W9-ATL-737

UNDERGROUND CLINICAL VIGNETTES

....

MICROBIOLOGY VOL. I

Classic Clinical Cases for
USMLE Step 1 Review [109 cases, 2nd ed]

VIKAS BHUSHAN, MD
University of California, San Francisco, Class of 1991
Series Editor, Diagnostic Radiologist

CHIRAG AMIN, MD
University of Miami, Class of 1996
Orlando Regional Medical Center, Resident in Orthopaedic Surgery

TAO LE, MD
University of California, San Francisco, Class of 1996
Yale-New Haven Hospital, Resident in Internal Medicine

JOSE M. FIERRO
La Salle University, Mexico City
Brookdale University Hospital, New York, Intern in Medicine/Pediatrics

HOANG NGUYEN
Northwestern University, Class of 2000

VISHAL PALL, MBBS
Government Medical College, Chandigarh, India, Class of 1996

©1999 by S2S Medical Publishing

NOTICE: The authors of this volume have taken care that the information contained herein is accurate and compatible with the standards generally accepted at the time of publication. Nevertheless, it is difficult to ensure that all the information given is entirely accurate for all circumstances. The publisher and authors do not guarantee the contents of this book and disclaim any liability, loss, or damage incurred as a consequence, directly or indirectly, of the use and application of any of the contents of this volume.

Distributed by Blackwell Science, Inc.
Editorial Office:
Commerce Place, 350 Main Street, Malden, Massachusetts 02148, USA

Distributors
USA
Blackwell Science, Inc.
Commerce Place
350 Main Street
Malden, Massachusetts 02148
(Telephone orders: 800-215-1000 or
781-388-8250;
fax orders: 781-388-8270)

Canada
Login Brothers Book Company
324 Saulteaux Crescent
Winnipeg, Manitoba, R3J 3T2
(Telephone orders: 204-224-4068;
Telephone: 800-665-1148; fax: 800-665-0103)

Australia
Blackwell Science Pty, Ltd.
54 University Street
Carlton, Victoria 3053
(Telephone orders: 03-9347-0300;
fax orders: 03-9349-3016)

Outside North America and Australia
Blackwell Science, Ltd.
c/o Marston Book Services, Ltd.
P.O. Box 269
Abingdon
Oxon OX14 4YN
England
(Telephone orders: 44-01235-465500;
fax orders: 44-01235-465555)

ISBN: 1-890061-16-6

Editor: Andrea Fellows
Typesetter: Vikas Bhushan using MS Word97
Printed and bound by Capital City Press

Printed in the United States of America
99 00 01 02 6 5 4 3 2

All rights reserved. No part of this book may be reproduced in any form or by any electronic or mechanical means, including information storage and retrieval systems, without permission in writing from the publisher, except by a reviewer who may quote brief passages in a review.

Contributors

....

SAMIR MEHTA
Temple University, Class of 2000

ALEA EUSEBIO
UCLA School of Medicine, Class of 2000

MARK TANAKA
UCSF School of Medicine, Class of 1999

RAJNI JUTLA
Cambridge Overseas Medical Training Programme, Class of 2001

Faculty Reviewer

....

WARREN LEVINSON, MD, PHD
Professor of Microbiology and Immunology, UCSF School of Medicine

Acknowledgments

....

Throughout the production of this book, we have had the support of many friends and colleagues. Special thanks to our business manager, Gianni Le Nguyen. For expert computer support, Tarun Mathur and Alex Grimm. For design suggestions, Sonia Santos and Elizabeth Sanders.

For editing, proofreading, and assistance across the vignette series, we collectively thank Carolyn Alexander, Henry E. Aryan, Natalie Barteneva, Sanjay Bindra, Julianne Brown, Hebert Chen, Arnold Chin, Yoon Cho, Karekin R. Cunningham, A. Sean Dalley, Sunit Das, Ryan Armando Dave, Robert DeMello, David Donson, Alea Eusebio, Priscilla A. Frase, Anil Gehi, Parul Goyal, Alex Grimm, Tim Jackson, Sundar Jayaraman, Aarchan Joshi, Rajni K. Jutla, Faiyaz Kapadi, Aaron S. Kesselheim, Sana Khan, Andrew Pin-wei Ko, Warren S. Krackov, Benjamin H.S. Lau, Scott Lee, Warren Levinson, Eric Ley, Ken Lin, Samir Mehta, Gil Melmed, Joe Messina, Vivek Nandkarni, Deanna Nobleza, Darin T. Okuda, Adam L. Palance, Sonny Patel, Ricardo Pietrobon, Riva L. Rahl, Aashita Randeria, Marilou Reyes, Diego Ruiz, Anthony Russell, Sanjay Sahgal, Sonal Shah, John Stulak, Lillian Su, Julie Sundaram, Rita Suri, Richa Varma, Amy Williams, Ashraf Zaman and David Zipf. Please let us know if your name has been missed or mispelled and we will be happy to make the change in the next edition.

Table of Contents

. . . .

CASE	SUBSPECIALTY	NAME
40	ID	Cytomegalovirus (CMV) Pneumonitis
41	ID	Diphtheria
42	ID	Echinococcosis
43	ID	Endotoxic Shock
44	ID	Epidemic Typhus (*Rickettsia prowazekii*)
45	ID	Epiglottitis (*H. influenzae*)
46	ID	Giardiasis
47	ID	Gonococcal Arthritis
48	ID	Gonorrhea
49	ID	Herpes Simplex (Type 2)
50	ID	Histoplasmosis
51	ID	Human Papillomavirus (HPV)
52	ID	Human T-Cell Leukemia Virus Type 1
53	ID	Infectious Mononucleosis (EBV)
54	ID	Legionella Pneumonia (Legionnaire's)
55	ID	Leishmaniasis
56	ID	Leprosy (Tuberculoid)
57	ID	Listeriosis
58	ID	Lyme Disease
59	ID	Lymphatic Filariasis
60	ID	Lymphogranuloma Venereum
61	ID	Malaria
62	ID	Measles
63	ID	Meningococcemia
64	ID	Mucormycosis
65	ID	Mumps
66	ID	Mycoplasma Pneumonia
67	ID	Nocardiosis
68	ID	Onchocerciasis
69	ID	Osteomyelitis
70	ID	Otitis Media
71	ID	*Pasteurella multocida*
72	ID	Plague
73	ID	Pneumococcal Pneumonia
74	ID	*Pneumocystis carinii* Pneumonia
75	ID	Pulmonary Tuberculosis
76	ID	Rabies
77	ID	Rubella - Congenital
78	ID	Rubella (German Measles)
79	ID	Scarlet Fever
80	ID	Schistosomiasis
81	ID	Shigellosis
82	ID	Sporotrichosis
83	ID	Streptococcal Pharyngitis
84	ID	Strongyloidiasis
85	ID	Subdiaphragmatic Abscess
86	ID	Syphilis - Congenital
87	ID	Syphilis - Primary

CASE	SUBSPECIALTY	NAME
88	ID	Syphilis - Secondary
89	ID	Tetanus
90	ID	Toxoplasmosis
91	ID	Trichinosis
92	ID	Tularemia
93	ID	Typhoid Fever (Enteric Fever)
94	ID	Varicella Zoster -Chickenpox
95	ID	Varicella Zoster -Shingles
96	ID	Whooping Cough
97	ID	Yellow Fever
98	Neurology	Bacterial Meningitis - Adult
99	Neurology	Bacterial Meningitis - Pediatric
100	Neurology	Cryptococcal Meningitis
101	Neurology	Cytomegalovirus (CMV) Retinitis
102	Neurology	Neurocysticercosis
103	Neurology	Poliomyelitis
104	Neurology	Syphilis - Tertiary
105	Urology	Acute Cystitis
106	Urology	Acute Pyelonephritis
107	Urology	Nongonococcal Urethritis
108	Urology	Orchitis
109	Urology	Urinary Tract Infection (UTI)

Preface to the Second Edition

. . . .

We are very pleased with the overwhelmingly positive reception of the first edition of our *Underground Clinical Vignettes* series. In the second editions we have fine-tuned nearly every case by incorporating corrections, enhancements and clarifications. These were based on feedback from the several thousand students who used the first editions.

We implemented two structural changes upon the request of many students:

♦ bi-directional cross-linking to appropriate High Yield Facts in the 1999 edition of *First Aid for the USMLE Step 1* (Appleton & Lange);

♦ case names have been moved to the bottom of the page and obvious references to the case name within the case description have been removed.

With this, we hope they'll emerge as a unique and well-integrated study tool that provides compact clinical correlations to basic science information.

We invite your corrections and suggestions for the next edition of this book. For the first submission of each factual correction or new vignette, you will receive a personal acknowledgement and a free copy of the revised book. We prefer that you submit corrections or suggestions via electronic mail to vbhushan@aol.com. Please include "Underground Vignettes" as the subject of your message. If you do not have access to e-mail, use the following mailing address: S2S Medical Publishing, 1015 Gayley Ave, Box 1113, Los Angeles, CA 90024 USA.

Preface to the First Edition

. . . .

This series was developed to address the increasing number of clinical vignette questions on the USMLE Step 1 and Step 2. It is designed to supplement and complement *First Aid for the USMLE Step 1* (Appleton & Lange).

Each book uses a series of approximately 100 "**supra-prototypical**" cases **as a way to condense testable facts and associations**. The clinical vignettes in this series are designed to incorporate as many testable facts as possible into a cohesive and memorable clinical picture. The vignettes represent composites drawn from general and specialty textbooks, reference books, thousands of USMLE style questions and the personal experience of the authors and reviewers.

Although each case tends to present all the signs, symptoms, and diagnostic findings for a particular illness, **patients generally will not present with such a "complete" picture either clinically or on the Step 1 exam**. Cases are not meant to simulate a potential real patient or an exam vignette. All the **boldfaced "buzzwords" are for learning purposes** and are not necessarily expected to be found in any one patient with the disease.

Definitions of selected important terms are placed within the vignettes in (= SMALL CAPS) in parentheses. Other parenthetical remarks often refer to the pathophysiology or mechanism of disease. The format should also help students learn to present cases succinctly during oral "bullet" presentations on clinical rotations. The cases are meant to be read as a condensed review, not as a primary reference.

The information provided in this book has been prepared with a great deal of thought and careful research. This book should not, however, be considered as your sole source of information. Corrections, suggestions and submissions of new cases are encouraged and will be acknowledged and incorporated in future editions.

Abbreviations

ABGs – arterial blood gases
ADP – adenosine diphosphate
AIDS – acquired immunodeficiency syndrome
ALT – alanine transaminase
Angio – angiography
ARDS – acute respiratory distress syndrome
ASO – anti-streptolysin O
AST – aspartate transaminase
ATLL – adult T-cell leukemia/lymphoma
BE – barium enema
cAMP – cyclic adenosine monophosphate
CBC – complete blood count
CML – chronic myelogenous leukemia
CMV - cytomegalovirus
CN – cranial nerve
CNS – central nervous system
CPK – creatine phosphokinase
CRP – C-reactive protein
CSF – cerebrospinal fluid
CT – computerized tomography
CXR – chest x-ray
DIC – disseminated intravascular coagulation
DTP – diphtheria/tetanus toxoid/pertussis
EBV – Epstein–Barr virus
ECG – electrocardiography
Echo - echocardiography
ECM – erythema chronicum migrans
EEG – electroencephalography
EGD – esophagogastroduodenoscopy
EIA – enzyme immunoassay
ELISA – enzyme-linked immunosorbent assay
EMG – electromyography
ERCP – endoscopic retrograde cholangiopancreatography
ESR – erythrocyte sedimentation rate
FNA – fine needle aspiration
FTA-ABS – fluorescent treponemal antibody absorption
G6PD – glucose-6-phosphate deficiency
HAV – hepatitis A virus
HBV – hepatitis B virus
HIDA – hepatoiminodiacetic acid [scan]
HIV – human immunodeficiency virus
HPI – history of present illness
HPV – human papillomavirus
HTLV – human T-cell leukemia virus
ID/CC – identification and chief complaint
IDDM – insulin-dependent diabetes mellitus
Ig – immunoglobulin
INH – isoniazid
IVP – intravenous pyelography

Abbreviations - continued

JVP – jugular venous pressure
KOH – potassium hydroxide
KUB – kidneys/ureter/bladder
LDH – lactate dehydrogenase
LP – lumbar puncture
Lytes – electrolytes
Mammo – mammography
MMR – measles/mumps/rubella
MR – magnetic resonance [imaging]
Nuc – nuclear medicine
PA – posteroanterior
PAS – periodic acid-Schiff
PBS – peripheral blood smear
PE – physical exam
PET – positron emission tomography
PFTs – pulmonary function tests
PML – progressive multifocal leukoencephalopathy
PMN – polymorphonuclear leukocyte
PT – prothrombin time
PTT – partial thromboplastin time
RES – reticuloendothelial system
RHD – rheumatic heart disease
RSV – respiratory syncytial virus
SBFT – small bowel follow-through [barium study]
SMX-TMP – sulfamethoxazole–trimethoprim
SSPE – subacute sclerosing panencephalitis
STD – sexually transmitted disease
TP-HA – *Treponema pallidum* hemagglutination assay
UA – urinalysis
UGI – upper GI [barium study]
US – ultrasound
V/Q – ventilation perfusion
VDRL – Venereal Disease Research Laboratory
VS – vital signs
WBC – white blood cell
XR – x-ray

ID/CC	A 35-year-old male complains of **fever, nonproductive cough,** and **chest pain.**
HPI	He states that the chest pain developed after he had a severe cold for one week. He describes the pain as **severe, crushing, and constant** over the anterior chest and adds that it **worsens with inspiration** and is **relieved by sitting up** and bending forward.
PE	VS: low-grade fever; sinus tachycardia. PE: triphasic **pericardial friction rub** (systolic and diastolic components followed by a third component in late diastole associated with atrial contraction); **elevated JVP;** inappropriate **increase in JVP with inspiration** (= KUSSMAUL'S SIGN); pulsus paradoxus may also be seen.
Labs	Moderately elevated transaminases and LDH; **elevated ESR; serum CPK-MB normal.** CBC: neutrophilic leukocytosis. ECG: **diffuse ST-segment elevation** (vs. myocardial infarction); **PR-segment depression.**
Imaging	Echo: **pericardial effusion.** CXR: apparent **cardiomegaly** (due to effusion).
Gross Pathology	In long-standing cases, pericardium may become fibrotic, scarred, and calcified.
Micro Pathology	Pericardial biopsy reveals signs of acute inflammation with increased leukocytes, vascularity, and deposition of fibrin.
Treatment	Analgesics for pain; steroids in resistant cases; indomethacin; surgical stripping of scarring in severe cases.
Discussion	Commonly idiopathic. Known infectious causes include **coxsackievirus A and B, tuberculosis,** staphylococcal or pneumococcal infection, amebiasis, or actinomycosis; noninfectious causes include chronic renal failure, **collagen-vascular disease** (systemic lupus erythematosus, scleroderma, and rheumatoid arthritis), neoplasms, myocardial infarction, and trauma. Long-term sequelae include chronic constrictive pericarditis.

ACUTE PERICARDITIS

ID/CC	A 25-year-old female complains of low-grade fever and myalgia of three weeks' duration.
HPI	She has a history of **rheumatic heart disease** (RHD). One month ago, she underwent a **dental extraction** and did not take the antibiotics that were prescribed for her.
PE	VS: fever. PE: pallor; small, peripheral hemorrhages with slight nodular character (= JANEWAY LESIONS); small, tender nodules on finger and toe pads (= OSLER'S NODES); subungual linear streaks (= SPLINTER HEMORRHAGES); petechial hemorrhages on conjunctiva, oral mucosa, and upper extremities; mild splenomegaly; apical diastolic murmur on cardiovascular exam; fundus exam shows oval retinal hemorrhages (= ROTH'S SPOTS).
Labs	CBC/PBS: normocytic, normochromic anemia. UA: microscopic hematuria. Growth of penicillin-sensitive *Streptococcus viridans* on five of six blood cultures.
Imaging	Echo: vegetations along atrial surface of **mitral valve.**
Gross Pathology	Embolism from vegetative growths on valves may embolize peripherally (left-sided) or to the lung (right-sided).
Micro Pathology	Bacteria form nidus of infection in previously scarred or damaged valves; bacteria divide unimpeded once infection takes hold with further deposition of fibrin and platelets; peripheral symptoms such as Osler's nodes are believed to result from deposition of immune complexes.
Treatment	IV beta-lactamase-resistant penicillin and gentamicin; bacteriostatic treatments ineffective.
Discussion	*Streptococcus viridans* is the most common cause of subacute infective endocarditis, while *S. aureus* is the most common cause of acute bacterial endocarditis. Prophylactic antibiotics should be given to all RHD patients before any dental procedure. The disease continues to be associated with a high mortality rate. **FIRST AID** p.247

SUBACUTE BACTERIAL ENDOCARDITIS

ID/CC	A 25-year-old male complains of increasing **shortness of breath** and **ankle edema** that have progressively worsened over the past two weeks.
HPI	He also complains of fatigue, palpitations, and low-grade fever. His symptoms **followed a severe URI.** He denies any history of joint pain or skin rash (vs. rheumatic fever).
PE	JVP elevated; pitting pedal edema; fine inspiratory crepitations heard at both lung bases; mild hepatosplenomegaly.
Labs	ASO titers not elevated. CBC: lymphocytosis. ECG: first-degree AV block. ESR elevated; increased titers of antibodies to **coxsackievirus** demonstrated in serum.
Imaging	CXR: **cardiomegaly** and **pulmonary edema.** Echo: **dilated cardiomyopathy with low ejection fraction.**
Gross Pathology	Dilated heart with foci of epicardial, myocardial, and endocardial petechial hemorrhages.
Micro Pathology	Endomyocardial biopsy reveals **diffuse infiltration by mononuclear cells,** predominantly lymphocytes; focal fibrosis.
Treatment	Manage congestive heart failure and arrhythmias; cardiac transplant in intractable cases.
Discussion	**Coxsackie B** is most often implicated. Nonviral causes of myocarditis include bacteria such as *Borrelia burgdorferi* (Lyme disease), parasites such as *Trypanosoma cruzi* (Chagas' disease), hypersensitivity reaction (systemic lupus erythematosus, drug reaction), radiation, and sarcoidosis; may also be idiopathic (giant cell myocarditis).

VIRAL MYOCARDITIS

ID/CC	A 7-year-old boy **develops intense pruritus** and **blistering of the skin** over his arms and legs.
HPI	On the previous day, he had gone on a picnic and had spent the day **playing in the bushes.** He has no prior history of a similar illness.
PE	Erythematous, **papulovesicular rash** over both arms and legs; **oozing and crusting;** numerous scattered scratch marks.
Labs	N/A
Imaging	N/A
Gross Pathology	N/A
Micro Pathology	N/A
Treatment	Topical and systemic **corticosteroids;** once the allergen is removed, symptoms usually resolve within 2–3 weeks.
Discussion	This child has **poison ivy, a delayed-type (IV) hypersensitivity reaction.** Contact dermatitis may also be due to irritants (e.g, diaper rash). If the irritant is not known, **patch testing** with a standard group of allergens can elucidate the diagnosis.

. . . .

CONTACT DERMATITIS

ID/CC	A **5-year-old** white male presents with golden-yellow, crusted lesions around his mouth and behind his ears.
HPI	He has a history of intermittent low-grade fever, frequent "nose picking," and purulent discharge from his lesions. He has no history of hematuria (due to increased risk of poststreptococcal glomerulonephritis).
PE	Characteristic **"honey-colored" crusted lesions** seen at **angle of mouth,** around nasal orifices, and behind ears.
Labs	**Gram-positive cocci in chains** (= STREPTOCOCCI) in addition to pus cells on Gram stain of discharge; beta-hemolytic streptococci (group A streptococci) on blood agar culture; ASO titer negative.
Imaging	N/A
Gross Pathology	Erythematous lesions surrounding natural orifices with whitish or yellowish purulent exudate and crust formation.
Micro Pathology	Inflammatory infiltrate of PMNs with varying degrees of necrosis.
Treatment	Cephalosporin, penicillin, or erythromycin if allergic.
Discussion	A highly communicable infectious disease, most often caused by group A streptococci, that occurs primarily in preschoolers and may predispose to glomerulonephritis. It occurs most commonly on the face (periorbital area), hands, and arms. *Staphylococcus aureus* may coexist or cause bullous impetigo; group B streptococcal impetigo may be seen in newborns.

IMPETIGO

ID/CC	A 30-year-old male homosexual visits his family doctor complaining of a nonpruritic **skin eruption** on his **upper limbs, trunk,** and **anogenital area.**
HPI	He has been **HIV positive** for about three years and admits to having continued unprotected intercourse.
PE	Multiple painless, pearly-white, dome-shaped, waxy, **umbilicated nodules** 2–5 mm in diameter on arms, trunk, and anogenital area; **palms and soles spared.**
Labs	N/A
Imaging	N/A
Gross Pathology	Firm, umbilicated nodules containing thick yellowish material.
Micro Pathology	Stained histologic sections confirm diagnosis with large **cytoplasmic inclusions** (= MOLLUSCUM BODIES) in material expressed from lesions.
Treatment	Lesions may resolve spontaneously or be removed by curettage, cryotherapy, or podophyllin; no antiviral drug or vaccine available.
Discussion	A benign, autoinoculable disease of children and young adults caused by a poxvirus (DNA virus), it is transmitted through sexual contact, close bodily contact, clothing, or towels. One of many opportunistic infections seen in AIDS patients (difficult to eradicate).

MOLLUSCUM CONTAGIOSUM

ID/CC	A 6-year-old male presents with fever, intense headache, myalgia, dry cough, and a **rash that began peripherally** but now involves the entire body, **including the palms and soles.**
HPI	The child lives in North Carolina and indicates that he was **bitten by an insect** a few weeks ago while playing in the woods near his home.
PE	VS: fever. PE: lethargy; ill appearance; **petechial rash** all over body, including palms and soles.
Labs	CBC: thrombocytopenia; prolonged bleeding and clotting time. Positive Hess' capillary test (= RUMPEL–LEEDE PHENOMENON); **positive** *Proteus* OX19 and OX2 **Weil–Felix reaction;** specific antibodies to *Rickettsia rickettsii* with positive complement fixation. UA: proteinuria; hematuria.
Imaging	N/A
Gross Pathology	Hemorrhagic necrosis in brain and kidneys; nodular formation in glia.
Micro Pathology	Inflammatory lymphocytic and plasma cell perivascular infiltration; endothelial edema with abundant rickettsiae; microthrombus formation **with necrotic vasculitis.**
Treatment	Chloramphenicol; **tetracycline.**
Discussion	*Rickettsia rickettsii* is the causative organism; *Dermacentor*, a **wood tick, is the vector;** tropism for endothelial cells. Ironically, Rocky Mountain spotted fever is endemic to the East Coast of the U.S. **FIRST AID** p.186

ID/CC	An **18-month-old** male is brought to the pediatrician following the appearance of an extensive skin rash.
HPI	Four days ago he suddenly developed a **very high fever** (40 C) with no other symptoms or signs. The fever continued for four days until the day of his admission, when it abruptly **disappeared, coinciding with the onset of the rash.**
PE	**Child looks well;** in no acute distress; **generalized rash** apparent as discrete 2- to 5-mm **rose-pink macules and papules on trunk, neck, and extremities** (face is spared); lesions blanch on pressure; no lymphadenopathy; splenomegaly may also be present.
Labs	CBC/PBS: WBCs variable; relative lymphocytosis with atypical lymphocytes.
Imaging	N/A
Gross Pathology	N/A
Micro Pathology	N/A
Treatment	Supportive; foscarnet.
Discussion	Also called **exanthem subitum;** caused by **human herpesvirus 6.** The most common exanthematous disease in infants two years of age or younger, and a frequent cause of **febrile convulsions.**

ROSEOLA INFANTUM

ID/CC	A **2-month-old** female infant presents with extensive **bullae** and large areas of denuded skin.
HPI	Her mother had suffered from **staphylococcal mastitis** one week ago.
PE	VS: fever. PE: large areas of red, painful, denuded skin on periorbital and peribuccal areas; flaccid bullae with **easy dislodgment of epidermis under pressure** (= NIKOLSKY'S SIGN); mucosal surfaces largely uninvolved.
Labs	Vesicle fluid sterile; *S. aureus* on blood culture.
Imaging	N/A
Gross Pathology	N/A
Micro Pathology	N/A
Treatment	IV penicillinase-resistant penicillin (e.g., methicillin, oxacillin). Treat with erythromycin if patient is allergic to penicillin.
Discussion	Caused by the effect of phage group 2 **staphylococcal exotoxin.**

SCALDED SKIN SYNDROME

ID/CC	A 30-year-old man presents with a bilateral **red pruritic** skin **eruption** in the **groin** area.
HPI	N/A
PE	Bilateral, **circular papulosquamous skin eruption** on erythematous base with **active**, advancing **peripheral (serpiginous) border** over scrotum and perineum.
Labs	Microscopic examination reveals long septate **hyphae on KOH** skin scrapings.
Imaging	N/A
Gross Pathology	N/A
Micro Pathology	N/A
Treatment	Topical antifungal agents (Whitfield's ointment, clotrimazole, miconazole); systemic therapy with oral griseofulvin, ketoconazole, or itraconazole in resistant cases.
Discussion	Tinea corporis (= COMMON RINGWORM) occurs sporadically; *Trichophyton rubrum* is the most common cause. The inflammatory form, which is usually localized to the limbs, chest, or back, is commonly caused by *Microsporum canis* or *Trichophyton mentagrophytes*. Ringworm of the scalp, known as tinea capitis, is commonly seen in children.

. . . .

TINEA CORPORIS (RINGWORM)

ID/CC	A 28-year-old male presents with a **red, pruritic skin eruption** on his trunk and his upper and lower limbs of a few hours' duration.
HPI	One day earlier, he was prescribed cotrimoxazole for a UTI. He has not experienced any dyspnea.
PE	Erythematous, warm, urticarial wheals (hives) seen over trunk, legs, and arms; no angioedema or respiratory distress.
Labs	CBC: leukocytosis with eosinophilia. No parasites revealed on stool exam.
Imaging	N/A
Gross Pathology	Linear or oval, **raised papules or plaque-like wheals** up to several centimeters in diameter.
Micro Pathology	Wide separation of dermal collagen fibers with dilatation of lymphatics and venules.
Treatment	Topical agents such as calamine lotion to reduce itching; corticosteroids; avoidance of causative agent (in this case, cotrimoxazole); H_1 and H_2 blockers.
Discussion	Mast cells and basophils are focal to urticarial reaction. When stimulated by certain immunologic or nonimmunologic mechanisms, storage granules in these cells release histamine and other mediators, such as kinins and leukotrienes. These agents produce the localized vasodilatation and transudation of fluid that characterize urticaria.

URTICARIA

ID/CC An 11-year-old white male presents with **jaundice** and **dark yellow urine** that has been present for the last several days.

HPI He also complains of nausea, vomiting, and malaise. For the past two weeks, he has also had a low-grade fever and mild abdominal pain. He recently returned from a **vacation in Mexico,** where he said he consumed a lot of **shellfish.**

PE Icterus; tender, firm hepatomegaly; no evidence of splenomegaly or free fluid in the peritoneal cavity.

Labs **Direct hyperbilirubinemia;** elevated serum transaminases (ALT > AST); modestly elevated alkaline phosphatase; prolonged PT; increased urinary urobilinogen and bilirubin; **positive IgM antibody to hepatitis A (HAV)** indicative of active HAV infection.

Imaging N/A

Gross Pathology May often appear normal.

Micro Pathology Multifocal hepatocellular necrosis with Councilman bodies; lymphocytic infiltrates around necrotic foci; loss of lobular architecture.

Treatment Supportive management; passive vaccination available.

Discussion Virus is shed 14–21 days before the onset of **jaundice;** patients are no longer infectious 21 days after clinical symptoms. Spread by **fecal–oral transmission;** endemic in areas where there are **contaminated water sources. No chronic-carrier state;** recovery takes place in 6–12 months. HAV is a naked, single-stranded RNA virus of the **picorna** family. A killed vaccine is available; passive immunization in the form of immune serum globulins is also available.
FIRST AID p.196

. . . .

HEPATITIS A INFECTION

ID/CC	A 25-year-old male medical student presents with **jaundice** and **dark yellow urine.**
HPI	He admits to having experienced an accidental **needle stick** two months ago, which he did not report. He also complains of nausea, low-grade fever, and loss of appetite.
PE	Icterus; tender, firm **hepatomegaly;** no evidence of ascites or splenomegaly.
Labs	**Direct hyperbilirubinemia;** elevated serum transaminases (ALT > AST); mildly elevated alkaline phosphatase; **HBsAg positive; IgM anti-HBc positive** (present during window period).
Imaging	US-Abdomen: hepatomegaly; increased echogenicity.
Gross Pathology	Liver may be enlarged, congested, or jaundiced; in fulminant cases of massive hepatic necrosis, liver becomes small, shrunken, and soft (acute yellow atrophy).
Micro Pathology	Liver biopsy reveals hepatocellular necrosis with **Councilman bodies** and ballooning degeneration; inflammation of portal areas with infiltration of mononuclear cells (small lymphocytes, plasma cells, eosinophils); prominence of Kupffer cells and bile ducts; cholestasis with bile plugs.
Treatment	Supportive care; follow-up to determine continued presence of HBsAg for at least six months as sign of chronic hepatitis; vaccine available for prevention.
Discussion	**Hepatitis B immune globulin** plus **hepatitis B vaccine** are recommended for parenteral or mucosal exposure to blood and for newborns of HBsAg-positive mothers. The infection is divided into the prodromal, icteric, and convalescent phases; **5% proceed to chronic hepatitis** with increased risk for cirrhosis and **hepatocellular carcinoma.** Unlike hepatitis A, hepatitis B has a long incubation period (three months). Hepatitis B virus is an enveloped, partially circular DNA virus of the **hepadna** family that contains a DNA-dependent DNA polymerase. The continued presence of HBsAg after infection has clinically resolved indicates a chronic carrier state. **FIRST AID** p.199

. . . .

HEPATITIS B INFECTION

ID/CC	A 30-year-old male is referred for an evaluation of **intermittent jaundice** over the past two years.
HPI	He also complains of diarrhea, skin rash, and weight loss. He received a **blood transfusion** one year ago, when he was injured in a motorcycle accident. He denies any IV drug use or any history of neuropsychiatric disorders in his family.
PE	**Icterus;** firm, **tender hepatomegaly;** splenomegaly; no evidence of ascites; no Kayser-Fleischer rings found on slit-lamp examination (vs. Wilson's disease).
Labs	Direct hyperbilirubinemia; markedly raised serum transaminase levels; **hepatitis B (HBV) serology negative;** enzyme immunoassay of antibodies to structural and nonstructural enzyme proteins of **hepatitis C (C200, C33c, C22-3) positive.**
Imaging	N/A
Gross Pathology	N/A
Micro Pathology	On liver biopsy, presence of ballooning degeneration; **portal inflammation with necrosis of hepatocytes within parenchyma** or immediately adjacent to portal areas (= "PIECEMEAL NECROSIS.").
Treatment	Alpha-2b-interferon; supportive management.
Discussion	Hepatitis C belongs to the **flavivirus** family and is currently the most important cause of **post-transfusion viral hepatitis;** 90% of cases involve percutaneous transmission. Greater than 50% of cases progress to chronic hepatitis, leading to cirrhosis in 20%. **FIRST AID** p.196

. . . .

HEPATITIS C INFECTION (CHRONIC ACTIVE HEPATITIS)

ID/CC	A 50-year-old alcoholic white male presents with **fever, abdominal pain,** and rapidly progressive distention of the abdomen.
HPI	He was diagnosed with **alcoholic cirrhosis** one month ago, when he was admitted to the hospital with jaundice and hematemesis.
PE	VS: fever. PE: icterus; on palpation, abdominal tenderness with guarding; fluid thrill and shifting dullness to percussion (due to **ascites**); **splenomegaly;** decreased bowel sounds.
Labs	CBC: **leukocytosis**. Ascitic fluid leukocyte count > 500/cc; PMNs (350/cc) elevated; ascitic proteins and glucose depressed; gram-negative bacilli in ascitic fluid; *E. coli* isolated in culture; elevated AST and ALT (AST > ALT).
Imaging	KUB: ground-glass haziness (due to ascites); no evidence of free air. US-Abdomen: cirrhotic shrunken liver; **ascites; splenomegaly; increased portal vein diameter and flow.** EGD: esophageal varices.
Gross Pathology	Fibrinopurulent exudate covering surface of peritoneum; fibrosis may lead to formation of adhesions.
Micro Pathology	PMNs and fibrin on serosal surfaces in various stages with presence of granulation tissue and fibrosis.
Treatment	Specific organism-sensitive antibiotics or empiric therapy for gram-negative aerobic bacilli and gram-positive cocci; supportive treatment for cirrhosis.
Discussion	The spontaneous or primary form of peritonitis occurs in patients with advanced chronic liver disease and concomitant ascites; *E. coli* is the most common cause of secondary peritonitis.

SPONTANEOUS BACTERIAL PERITONITIS

ID/CC   A 56-year-old white male complains of **diarrhea** and bloating for **several months** along with ankle swelling.

HPI   He also complains of memory loss, fever, **arthritis** in the knees and hands, and **weight loss.**

PE   VS: fever. PE: thin, gaunt male; muscle wasting; swollen, tender right wrist and ankle; axillary and femoral lymphadenopathy; ecchymoses of chest and arms.

Labs   CBC/PBS: macrocytic, hypochromic anemia; hypoalbuminemia; **increased fecal fat** (steatorrhea).

Imaging   UGI/SBFT: nonspecific dilatation of small bowel.

Gross Pathology   Atrophy of intestinal mucosa; inflammatory infiltrate in synovia of joints.

Micro Pathology   Small bowel biopsy reveals **characteristic macrophages** containing bacilli with **PAS** reagent staining; characteristic gram-positive *Actinomycete* bacilli in macrophages, PMNs, and epithelial cells of lamina propria; dilated lymphatics; flattening of intestinal villi.

Treatment   Bactrim or ceftriaxone for one year.

Discussion   Caused by infection with *Tropheryma whippelii;* produces **malabsorption** of fat-soluble vitamins, protein, iron, folic acid, and vitamin B_{13}.

. . . .

WHIPPLE'S DISEASE

ID/CC	A 19-year-old male has **recurrent attacks** of bilateral **periorbital and hand swelling** coupled with **respiratory difficulty that lasts up to 24 hours** and often requires hospitalization.
HPI	His **father** and his **aunt** both suffer from a **similar illness.**
PE	Physical examination unremarkable.
Labs	**Decreased C4** (best screening test); **decreased C1 inhibitor** (confirmatory test) and C2; normal C3; normal IgE.
Imaging	N/A
Gross Pathology	N/A
Micro Pathology	N/A
Treatment	Synthetic androgens (e.g., danazol), fresh frozen plasma.
Discussion	Inherited as an **autosomal-dominant** trait; **death** may result from **laryngeal edema.** Also known as hereditary angioedema. **FIRST AID** p.207

ID/CC A 3-year-old **albino** male is referred to a specialist for an evaluation of a suspected immune deficiency.

HPI His parents report **recurrent** respiratory, skin, and oral **infections with gram-negative and gram-positive** organisms. He also has a history of bruising easily.

PE **Partial albinism;** light-brown hair with silvery tint; **nystagmus; photophobia** on eye reflex exam; chronic gingivitis and periodontitis; purpuric patches over areas of repeated minimal trauma; mild hepatomegaly; no lymphadenopathy.

Labs CBC/PBS: **decreased neutrophil count** with normal platelet count; **large cytoplasmic granules** (= GIANT LYSOSOMES) in WBCs on Wright-stained peripheral blood smears. Prolonged bleeding time; impaired platelet aggregation; normal clotting time and PTT; normal nitroblue tetrazolium test.

Imaging N/A

Gross Pathology N/A

Micro Pathology N/A

Treatment Largely supportive; ascorbic acid, prophylactic antibiotics, acyclovir.

Discussion An **autosomal-recessive** disorder due to a **defect in polymerization of microtubules in leukocytes,** causing impairment of chemotaxis, phagocytosis, and formation of phagolysosomes. Patients with this disorder usually present with **recurrent pyogenic staphylococcal and streptococcal infections.** FIRST AID p.209

. . . .

CHÉDIAK–HIGASHI SYNDROME

ID/CC	A **2-year-old male** is admitted to the hospital for evaluation of a suspected immune disorder.
HPI	He has a history of **recurrent fungal** diaper rashes and **staphylococcal cervical furunculosis** requiring multiple incisions and drainage in addition to antibiotics. His mother also reports chronic diarrhea and a prior perianal fistula.
PE	Cervical lymphadenopathy; mild hepatomegaly and splenomegaly; no pallor, purpuric patches, or sternal tenderness.
Labs	CBC/PBS: **neutrophilic leukocytosis.** Elevated ESR; normal serum immunoglobulins; **absence of respiratory burst** (negative nitroblue tetrazolium test and chemoluminescence assay); negative Mantoux test.
Imaging	CXR: hilar lymphadenopathy. US-Abdomen: hepatosplenomegaly; hepatic and splenic nodular lesions (due to granulomas).
Gross Pathology	N/A
Micro Pathology	Characteristic granuloma formation with phagocytes, giant cells, and occasional histiocytes in lymph nodes, liver, spleen, and lungs.
Treatment	Long-term SMX–TMP prophylaxis, gamma-interferon.
Discussion	Most commonly an **X-linked** disorder of neutrophil function (may have variable inheritance patterns); due to a **deficiency of NADPH oxidase.** Neutrophils of affected patients demonstrate normal chemotaxis, degranulation, and phagocytosis but cannot use oxygen-dependent myeloperoxidase system for microbial killing, making patients susceptible to recurrent staphylococcal infections. **FIRST AID** p.209

CHRONIC GRANULOMATOUS DISEASE

ID/CC	A 25-year-old **white** female is referred to an internist by her family doctor for a workup of **recurrent sinusitis**, chronic otitis media, one episode of **pneumonia** that required hospitalization, and recurrent bouts of watery **diarrhea.**
HPI	She has seen an allergy specialist for several years and has received desensitization shots for **multiple allergies,** including pollen, dust, and cat hair.
PE	Normal except for **hypopigmented spots on neck and arms** (= VITILIGO).
Labs	**Markedly decreased serum IgA; normal IgG and IgM.**
Imaging	XR-Sinus: opacification of paranasal sinuses (due to chronic sinusitis).
Gross Pathology	N/A
Micro Pathology	N/A
Treatment	Largely supportive; antibiotic therapy; try to **avoid blood or plasma transfusion** (anaphylaxis or serum sickness due to presence of antibodies to IgA).
Discussion	The **most common congenital immunodeficiency.** Diarrhea is usually caused by *Giardia lamblia;* recurrent sinopulmonary infections are caused by *S. pneumoniae, H. influenzae,* or *S. aureus;* associated with an increased incidence of allergies and autoimmune diseases. Selective IgA deficiency may be due to a specific defect in isotype switching. **FIRST AID** p.209

ID/CC	A 7-month-old **male** is admitted for a workup of **recurrent upper respiratory tract and skin infections** of several months' duration.
HPI	His parents state that he has had recurrent URIs, one episode of *H. influenzae* **pneumonia,** and severe otitis media.
PE	Low weight and height for chronological age; chronic bilateral suppurative otitis media; **asymmetric arthritis** of knees; **no tonsillar tissue** seen; no lymphadenopathy or hepatosplenomegaly.
Labs	**Panhypogammaglobulinemia: very low** IgG; IgA and IgM undetectable.
Imaging	N/A
Gross Pathology	N/A
Micro Pathology	N/A
Treatment	Parenteral gamma globulin; monitor pulmonary function to guard against chronic lung disease.
Discussion	An X-linked disease (manifests **only in males**) characterized by a **selective B-cell defect** with **recurrent bacterial infections.** Also known as **Bruton's disease,** it is due to a genetic defect in tyrosine kinase receptor found on antibody precursors, resulting in impaired maturation and development of antibodies. **FIRST AID** p.209

ID/CC	A 7-year-old male is brought to his family physician complaining of a **thick yellowish discharge in his eyes that prevents him from opening his eyes in the morning;** for the past few days, his eyes have been **blood-red, painful,** and **watery.** His eye pain is exacerbated by exposure to light (= PHOTOPHOBIA).
HPI	Three of his classmates and a neighbor had a similar episode about seven days ago (suggesting a **local epidemic** of such cases).
PE	VS: no fever. PE: **normal visual acuity; erythematous palpebral conjunctiva;** watery eyes; **remains of thick mucus** found on inner canthal area; no corneal infiltrate on slit-lamp exam; normal anterior chamber; **mild preauricular lymphadenopathy.**
Labs	Stained conjunctival smears reveal **lymphocytes,** giant cells, **neutrophils,** and bacteria.
Imaging	N/A
Gross Pathology	N/A
Micro Pathology	N/A
Treatment	Topical antimicrobial eye drops; cool compresses; minimize contact with others to avoid spread; avoid use of topical steroid preparations, as these can exacerbate bacterial and viral eye infections.
Discussion	Conjunctivitis is a common disease of childhood that is mostly viral **(adenovirus)** and self-limiting; it occurs in epidemics, and secondary bacterial infections (staphylococci and streptococci) may result. Visual acuity is not affected.

. . . .

ACUTE CONJUNCTIVITIS

ID/CC	An **8-year-old** female presents with pain and swelling of her knee joints, elbows, and lower limbs along with **fever** for the past two weeks; she also complains of shortness of breath (= DYSPNEA) on exertion.
HPI	The patient had a **sore throat two weeks ago.**
PE	VS: fever. PE: **blanching, ring-shaped erythematous rash over trunk and proximal extremities** (= ERYTHEMA MARGINATUM); **subcutaneous nodules** at occiput and below extensor tendons in elbow; **swelling with redness of both knee joints and elbows** (= POLYARTHRITIS); painfully restricted movement; pedal edema; increased JVP; high-frequency apical systolic murmur with radiation to axillae **(mitral valve insufficiency due to carditis)**; bilateral fine inspiratory basal crepitant rales; mild, tender hepatomegaly.
Labs	CBC: leukocytosis. *Streptococcus pyogenes* on throat swab; markedly **elevated ASO titers; elevated ESR; elevated C-reactive protein (CRP)**; negative blood culture. ECG: **prolonged P-R interval.**
Imaging	CXR: cardiomegaly; increased pulmonary vascular markings. Echo: vegetations over mitral valve with regurgitation.
Gross Pathology	Acute form characterized by **endo-, myo-, and pericarditis** (= PANCARDITIS); chronic form characterized by fibrous scarring with calcification and mitral stenosis with verrucous fibrin deposits.
Micro Pathology	Myocardial muscle fiber necrosis enmeshed in collagen; characteristic finding is fibrinoid necrosis surrounded by **perivascular accumulation of mononuclear inflammatory cells (= ASCHOFF CELLS).**
Treatment	Aspirin and corticosteroids; penicillin or erythromycin.
Discussion	A sequela of infection with group A, beta-hemolytic streptococcus; causes **autoimmune** damage to several organs, mostly the heart. The systemic effects of acute rheumatic fever are immune mediated and are secondary to cross-reactivity of host antistreptococcal antibodies. **FIRST AID** p.247

ACUTE RHEUMATIC FEVER

ID/CC	A 35-year-old woman complains of fever and **pain in the face** and **upper teeth** (maxillary sinus), especially while leaning forward.
HPI	She has had a chronic cough, **nasal congestion, and discharge** for the past few months.
PE	VS: fever. PE: halitosis; greenish-yellow **postnasal discharge;** bilateral **boggy nasal mucosa;** bilateral percussion tenderness and **erythema over zygomatic arch; clouding of sinuses by transillumination;** dental and cranial nerve exams normal.
Labs	Nasal cultures reveal *S. pneumoniae.*
Imaging	CT-Sinus: partial opacification of maxillary sinus with air–fluid level.
Gross Pathology	Erythematous and edematous nasal mucosa.
Micro Pathology	Presence of organisms and leukocytes in mucosa.
Treatment	Oral decongestants; amoxicillin.
Discussion	Other pathogens include other streptococci, *H. influenzae,* and *Moraxella.* The obstruction of ostia in the anterior ethmoid and middle meatal complex by retained secretions, mucosal edema, or polyps promotes sinusitis.

7) flu
S. pneumo
M. cat

sinusitis, otitis media, pneumonia

. . . .

ACUTE SINUSITIS

ID/CC   A 48-year-old missionary who has lived in Cameroon, **West Africa,** for 20 years is airlifted home because of **lethargy, nuchal rigidity, persistent headache, and drowsiness** that have not responded to antibiotics and supportive treatment.

HPI   He states that over the years he has been bitten in the neck several times by a mutumutu, or **tsetse fly** (= *GLOSSINA PALPALIS*). He has also had intermittent, generalized erythematous rashes accompanied by fever.

PE   Alert but somewhat **incoherent and confused;** sometimes delusional; nuchal rigidity and **tremors of face and lips;** splenomegaly; generalized **rubbery, painless lymphadenopathy,** predominantly in posterior neck and supraclavicular areas (= WINTERBOTTOM'S SIGN).

Labs   PBS/LP: hypercellular, **trypanosomal** forms present; lymphocytes in CSF. **Elevated IgM.**

Imaging   N/A

Gross Pathology   Chancre with erythema and induration at bite site; chancre resolves spontaneously; spleen and lymph nodes enlarged during systemic stage; leptomeninges enlarged during CNS involvement.

Micro Pathology   Skin: edema, mononuclear cell inflammation, organisms, and endothelial proliferation; spleen and lymph nodes: histiocytic hyperplasia; CNS: mononuclear cell meningoencephalitis.

Treatment   Suramin; pentamidine.

Discussion   Also called **sleeping sickness,** it is a systemic disease endemic to Africa whose chronic form causes a meningoencephalitis. Caused by the flagellated protozoan *Trypanosoma brucei gambiense* or *Trypanosoma brucei rhodesiense*; transmitted by the tsetse fly.

. . . .

AFRICAN TRYPANOSOMIASIS

ID/CC	A 17-year-old boy presents with **itchy eyes,** nasal stuffiness, increased lacrimation, **sneezing,** and a **watery nasal discharge.**
HPI	He has had similar episodes in the past that have corresponded with **changing of the seasons.** His mother is known to have bronchial asthma.
PE	VS: no fever. PE: pallor; **boggy nasal mucosa; nasal polyps present;** conjunctiva congested; no exudate.
Labs	Conjunctival and nasal smear demonstrates presence of **eosinophils;** no bacteria on Gram stain; no neutrophils.
Imaging	N/A
Gross Pathology	Nasal mucosa hyperemic and swollen with fluid transudation.
Micro Pathology	Local tissue inflammation and dysfunction of upper airway because of type I, IgE-mediated hypersensitivity response.
Treatment	Oral decongestants with intranasal corticosteroids; intranasal cromolyn sodium, especially before anticipated contact with allergen.
Discussion	Commonly caused by exposure to **pollens;** symptoms are mediated by the release of vasoactive and chemotactic mediators from mast cells and basophils (e.g., histamine and leukotrienes) with IgE surface receptors.

ALLERGIC RHINITIS (HAY FEVER)

ID/CC	A 45-year-old male Peace Corps volunteer who recently spent two years in rural Mexico complains of a **spiking fever,** malaise, headache, and **right upper quadrant abdominal pain.**
HPI	He admits to having had **bloody diarrhea with mucus** (= DYSENTERY) and tenesmus that disappeared with some pills that he took several months ago.
PE	VS: fever (39.6 C). PE: pallor; slight jaundice; tender **3+ hepatomegaly** with no rebound tenderness; pain on fist percussion of right lower ribs.
Labs	CBC: leukocytosis with neutrophilia. Amebic cysts in stool specimen (not concurrent with abscess); positive serology for antibodies to *Entamoeba histolytica.*
Imaging	CXR: elevation of right hemidiaphragm; small right pleural effusion. CT/US: cavitating lesion in **right lobe of liver** (due to abscess).
Gross Pathology	Multiple mucosal ulcers, slightly raised and covered with shaggy exudate; enlarged liver with **one large abscess** on right lobe containing chocolate-colored pus; abscess may rupture and spread to lungs, brain, or other organs.
Micro Pathology	Sterile pus; ameba may be obtained from periphery of lesion.
Treatment	Metronidazole; needle evacuation; surgery in case of treatment failure or rupture.
Discussion	Prior travel to endemic areas, plus a triad of fever, hepatomegaly, and right upper quadrant pain, are hallmarks of hepatic liver abscess.

· ·

AMEBIC LIVER ABSCESS

ID/CC   A 30-year-old male goes to the emergency room because of **dyspnea,** cyanosis, hemoptysis, and chest pain.

HPI   He has had a high fever, malaise, and a **nonproductive cough** for one week. The patient is a **sheep farmer** who remembers having been treated for **dark black skin lesions** in the past.

PE   VS: fever. PE: dyspnea; cyanosis; bilateral rales heard over lungs.

Labs   CBC: normal. Negative blood and sputum cultures; diagnosis of anthrax confirmed by fourfold increase in indirect microhemagglutination titer.

Imaging   CXR: mediastinal widening. CT-Chest: evidence of **"hemorrhagic mediastinitis."**

Gross Pathology   Patchy consolidation; vesicular papules covered by **black eschar.**

Micro Pathology   Lungs show fibrinous exudate with many organisms but few PMNs.

Treatment   Isolate and treat with IV penicillin G.

Discussion   Caused by infection with *Bacillus anthracis.* A cell-free anthrax vaccine is available to protect those employed in industries associated with a high risk of anthrax transmission (farmers, veterinarians, tannery or wool workers).

Gram + rods

spores {
Bacillus   anthracis
      cereus
Clostridium   botulinum
      tetani
      perfringens
      difficile

Corynebacterium diptheria
Listeria   monocytogenes.

. . . .

ANTHRAX

ID/CC A 38-year-old male receiving cytotoxic **chemotherapy** (immunosuppressed) for acute leukemia presents with **pleuritic chest pain,** hemoptysis, **fever,** and chills.

HPI He also complains of dyspnea, tachypnea, and a **productive cough.**

PE VS: fever. PE: severe respiratory distress; bilateral rales heard over lungs.

Labs CBC: severe **neutropenia.** Negative blood and sputum culture for bacteria.

Imaging CXR: necrotizing bronchopneumonia; multiple nodular infiltrates with cavitating lesion frequently crossing lung fissures (= FUNGUS BALL).

Gross Pathology **Necrotizing bronchopneumonia;** abscesses.

Micro Pathology Lung biopsy identifies *Aspergillus* with septate, acutely branching hyphae (visualized by silver stains); necrotizing inflammation; vascular thrombi with hyphae (due to **blood vessel invasion**).

Treatment Amphotericin B with flucytosine; lobectomy for fungus ball.

Discussion The most lethal form of infection, invasive aspergillosis, is seen primarily in severely immunocompromised individuals, i.e., patients with **AIDS**; patients with prolonged, **severe neutropenia** following cytotoxic chemotherapy; patients with **chronic granulomatous disease**; and patients receiving **glucocorticoids** and other **immunosuppressive drugs** (e.g., transplant recipients). **FIRST AID** p.189

no NADPH oxidase in PMN's → Staph infxn.

ASPERGILLOSIS

ID/CC	A 25-year-old male presents with sudden-onset **double vision** (= DIPLOPIA), **dry mouth, weakness, dysarthria,** and **dysphagia.**
HPI	He has no previous history of episodic weakness or of dog or tick bites (vs. myasthenia gravis, rabies, or Lyme disease). Last night, he ate some **home-canned food.**
PE	VS: no fever. PE: patient alert; ptosis; bilateral **third and tenth cranial nerve palsy;** symmetric **flaccid paralysis** of all four limbs; deep tendon reflexes reduced; no sensory loss seen; decreased bowel sounds.
Labs	Botulinum toxin detected in patient's serum and canned-food sample with specific antiserum.
Imaging	N/A
Gross Pathology	N/A
Micro Pathology	N/A
Treatment	Antitoxin; close monitoring of respiratory status; intubation for respiratory failure.
Discussion	Characterized by gradual return of muscle strength in most cases. Botulinum toxin is a zinc metalloprotease that cleaves specific components of synaptic vesicle docking and fusion complexes, thus **inhibiting the release of acetylcholine at the neuromuscular junction.** The disease in adults is due to **ingestion of the toxin** rather than to bacterial infection. Botulism is also seen in infants secondary to the ingestion of *Clostridium botulinum* spores in **honey.**

. . . .

BOTULISM

ID/CC	A **7-month-old** girl is brought to the pediatric clinic with **wheezing,** respiratory difficulty, and nasal congestion of three hours' duration.
HPI	She has had rhinorrhea, fever, and cough and had been sneezing for two days prior to her visit to the clinic.
PE	VS: **tachypnea.** PE: **nasal flaring;** mild central **cyanosis;** accessory muscle use during respiration; hyperexpansion of chest; expiratory and inspiratory wheezes; **rhonchi** over both lung fields.
Labs	CBC/PBS: relative **lymphocytosis.** ABGs: **hypoxemia with mild hypercapnia. Respiratory syncytial virus (RSV)** demonstrated on viral culture of throat swab.
Imaging	CXR: **hyperinflation;** segmental **atelectasis; interstitial infiltrates.**
Gross Pathology	N/A
Micro Pathology	N/A
Treatment	Humidified oxygen, bronchodilators, aerosolized **ribavirin.**
Discussion	**RSV is the most common cause of bronchiolitis in infants** under two years of age; other viral causes include parainfluenza, influenza, and adenovirus.

BRONCHIOLITIS

ID/CC   A 28-year-old white male visits his family doctor complaining of acute **pain in both hip joints** together with weakness, backache, myalgias, arthralgias, and **undulating fever** of **two months' duration**; this morning he woke up with pain in his right testicle.

HPI   For the past three years he has worked at the largest dairy farm in his state. He enjoys **drinking "crude" milk.**

PE   VS: fever. PE: pallor; marked pain on palpation of sacroiliac joints; mild splenomegaly; generalized lymphadenopathy.

Labs   CBC: lymphocytosis with normal WBC count. Positive agglutination titer (> 1:160); rising serologic titer over time; small gram-negative rod *Brucella abortus* on blood culture.

Imaging   N/A

Gross Pathology   Lymphadenopathy and splenomegaly; hepatomegaly rare.

Micro Pathology   Granulomatous foci in spleen, liver, and lymph nodes, with proliferation of macrophages; epithelioid and giant cells may be seen.

Treatment   Combination therapy with doxycycline or SMX–TMP and rifampin or streptomycin.

Discussion   Also called Malta fever, a microbial disease of animals, it is caused by several species of *Brucella*, a gram-negative, aerobic coccobacillus, and is transmitted to humans through the drinking of contaminated milk or direct contact with animal tissues. The clinical picture is often vague; thus, a high index of suspicion may be necessary for diagnosis.

undulating fever

. . . .

BRUCELLOSIS

ID/CC	A 49-year-old morbidly **obese, diabetic** woman presents with **pruritus in the skin folds** beneath her breasts.
HPI	She admits to having this problem chronically, especially in the warm summer months, when she perspires more heavily.
PE	Superficially **denuded, beefy red areas** beneath breasts with satellite vesicopustules and **whitish curd-like concretions** on surface.
Labs	Clusters of **budding cells with short hyphae** seen under high-power lens after skin scales have been put in 10% KOH; *Candida albicans* isolated in Sabouraud's medium.
Imaging	N/A
Gross Pathology	Rash has whitish-creamy pseudomembrane that covers an erythematous surface.
Micro Pathology	Yeast invades superficial layers of epithelium.
Treatment	Keep affected areas dry; clotrimazole locally.
Discussion	Other superficial areas of infection include the oral mucosa (thrush), vaginal mucosa (vaginitis), and esophagus (GI candidiasis). Systemic invasive candidiasis may be seen with immunosuppression, in patients receiving **chronic broad-spectrum antibiotics,** in AIDS patients, or in those receiving hyperalimentation. **FIRST AID** p.188, 189

CANDIDIASIS

ID/CC An 8-year-old white female enters the emergency room complaining of headache, malaise, and bipalpebral **swelling of the right eye.**

HPI She recently returned from a year-long stay in **Brazil,** where her father works as a logger in the Amazon **forest.** Over the past week she had a high fever, which was treated at home as malaria.

PE VS: fever (39 C); tachycardia. PE: right eyelid swollen shut (= ROMAÑA'S SIGN); markedly hyperemic conjunctiva; **ipsilateral retroauricular and cervical lymph nodes;** hepatosplenomegaly.

Labs PBS: **trypanosomes on thick blood smear.** ECG: right bundle-branch block; ventricular extrasystoles.

Imaging N/A

Gross Pathology Encapsulated, nodular area (= CHAGOMA) or Romaña's sign may be seen at point of entry, commonly face; can lead to life-threatening arrhythmias and heart block.

Micro Pathology Intense neutrophilic infiltrate with abundant macrophages at site of entry; myocardial necrosis with mononuclear cell infiltration; denervation of myenteric gut plexus.

myocardial pseudocyst

Treatment Nifurtimox for acute disease.

Discussion A parasitic disease that is restricted to the Americas (endemic in South and Central America), it is produced by *Trypanosoma cruzi,* a thin, undulating flagellated protozoan; it is transmitted by contamination of a **reduviid bug** bite with injection of its feces. Also known as American trypanosomiasis. Long-standing cases show myocardial involvement with **dilated cardiomyopathy** and apical aneurysm formation and may also show **megaesophagus or megacolon.**

. . . .

CHAGAS' DISEASE

ID/CC	A 30-year-old man has sudden severe, **profuse (several liters per day) watery diarrhea, protracted vomiting,** and **abdominal pain.**
HPI	He has just returned from a trip to **rural India.**
PE	**Severe dehydration;** low urine output; generalized mild abdominal tenderness with no signs of peritoneal irritation; stools have characteristic **"rice-water" appearance;** no blood or mucus in stools.
Labs	Stool culture reveals gram-negative rods with **"darting motility";** **O1 antigen detected;** *Vibrio cholerae* isolated on culture media; serum chloride levels decreased; serum sodium levels increased.
Imaging	N/A
Gross Pathology	N/A
Micro Pathology	N/A
Treatment	**Vigorous rehydration** therapy with oral and/or IV fluids; tetracycline.
Discussion	A heat-labile exotoxin produced by *Vibrio cholerae* that acts by permanently **stimulating G_s protein via ADP ribosylation,** resulting in activation of **intracellular adenylate cyclase,** which in turn increases cAMP levels and produces **secretory diarrhea.**

↑cAMP
Secretory diarrhea

tetracycline
VACUUM your BR

Vibrio
Acne
Chlamydia
Ureaplasma
Mycoplasma?
Borrelia
Ricketsia

CHOLERA

ID/CC A 19-year-old migrant worker from the **southwestern U.S.** is brought to the family doctor complaining of **cough, pleuritic chest pain, fever,** and malaise.

HPI He also complains of a backache and headache along with an **erythematous skin rash** (due to hypersensitivity reaction) in his lower limbs.

PE VS: fever; tachypnea. PE: central trachea; coarse, crepitant rales over both lung bases; tender, **erythematous nodules over shins** (= ERYTHEMA NODOSUM); periarticular swelling of knees and ankles.

Labs **Positive skin test with coccidioidin; dimorphic fungi** (hyphae in soil; spherules in body tissue), *Coccidioides immitis* on silver stain and sputum culture. CBC/PBS: eosinophilia.

Imaging CXR: nodular infiltrates and thin-walled cavities in both lower lungs.

Gross Pathology **Caseating granulomas;** often subpleural and in lower lobes; necrosis and cavitation may also be present.

Micro Pathology Silver-stained tissue sections show spherules filled with endospores.

Treatment Amphotericin B.

Discussion Endemic in the southwestern U.S.; produced by *Coccidioides immitis*. Transmitted by **inhalation of arthrospores.**
FIRST AID p.188

arthrospores form by fragmentation of hyphae

· ·

COCCIDIOIDOMYCOSIS

ID/CC	A 20-year-old male presents with a **runny nose, nasal congestion, sore throat, headache, and sneezing.**
HPI	He notes that his wife currently has similar symptoms.
PE	VS: mild fever. PE: rhinorrhea; congested and inflamed posterior pharyngeal wall; no lymphadenopathy.
Labs	Routine tests normal; routine throat swab staining and culture negative for bacteria.
Imaging	N/A
Gross Pathology	Nasal membranes edematous and erythematous with watery discharge.
Micro Pathology	Mononuclear inflammation of mucosa; focal desquamation.
Treatment	Symptomatic.
Discussion	Colds occur 2–3 times a year in the average person in the United States; the peak incidence is in the winter months. **Rhinoviruses** account for the majority of viral URIs, followed by coronaviruses. Spread occurs by **respiratory droplets** and **direct contact.** **FIRST AID** p.198

. . . .

COMMON COLD (VIRAL RESPIRATORY INFECTION)

ID/CC	A 30-year-old man with **AIDS** presents with chronic, recurrent **profuse, nonbloody, watery diarrhea.**
HPI	The diarrhea has recurred over the past two months with intermittent cramping, and previous treatments have not been effective.
PE	VS: no fever. PS: moderate **dehydration;** thin; generalized lymphadenopathy.
Labs	**Acid-fast** staining demonstrates oocysts of *Cryptosporidium* in fresh stool.
Imaging	N/A
Gross Pathology	Intestinal mucosa appears normal.
Micro Pathology	Blunting of intestinal villi; mixed inflammatory cell infiltrates with eosinophils in lamina propria; organisms visible on brush borders.
Treatment	No treatment found effective; supportive management with maintenance of fluids and nutrition.
Discussion	*Cryptosporidium parvum* infection presents as acute diarrhea in malnourished children and as severe diarrhea in immunocompromised patients (part of HIV wasting syndrome); the disease is mild and self-limiting in immune-competent patients. **FIRST AID** p.203

. . . .

CRYPTOSPORIDIOSIS

ID/CC   A newborn baby is referred to the pediatrician for further evaluation of an unusually **small head,** low birth weight, and an extensive **erythematous rash.**

HPI   **Intrauterine growth retardation** was prenatally diagnosed on ultrasound. The child's **mother had a flulike** episode during the **first trimester** of her pregnancy.   *cmv*

PE   Small for gestational age; generalized hypotonia with sluggish neonatal reflexes; extensive **"pinpoint" petechial skin rash** (= MULBERRY MUFFIN RASH); **microcephaly; chorioretinitis;** mild **icterus; hepatosplenomegaly; sensorineural hearing loss** in right ear.

Labs   CBC/PBS: mild thrombocytopenia. Moderately elevated direct serum bilirubin and transaminases. UA: cells in urine found to have large **intranuclear inclusions** (= "OWL'S EYE" INCLUSIONS); cytomegalovirus isolated on tissue culture.

Imaging   XR/CT-Head: periventricular calcifications; microcephaly.

Gross Pathology   N/A

Micro Pathology   N/A

Treatment   Ganciclovir (only for immunocompromised patients).

Discussion   A congenital herpesvirus infection involving the CNS with eye and ear damage; a common cause of mental retardation.

· ·

CYTOMEGALOVIRUS - CONGENITAL

ID/CC	A 13-year-old white female visits her pediatrician complaining of **fever**, severe **dyspnea**, and a **dry cough.**
HPI	She was recently diagnosed with acute lymphocytic leukemia, for which she received a **bone marrow** transplant. She is currently on **immunosuppressive therapy.**
PE	VS: fever; **tachypnea.** PE: pallor; **crepitant rales** over both lung fields; mild cyanosis; no hepatosplenomegaly.
Labs	CBC/PBS: anemia; leukopenia. ABGs: **hypoxemia.** No organism in induced sputum stained with Gram, Giemsa, ZN, and methenamine silver.
Imaging	CXR: diffuse, bilateral interstitial infiltrates.
Gross Pathology	**Interstitial pneumonitis;** hepatitis.
Micro Pathology	Characteristic **intranuclear inclusions with surrounding halo** (= OWL'S- OR BULL'S-EYE CELLS) on transbronchial lung biopsy.
Treatment	**Ganciclovir** (CMV is resistant to acyclovir).
Discussion	An enveloped, double-stranded DNA virus belonging to the herpesvirus group; the most common cause of pneumonia and death in **bone marrow transplant patients.** It is also common in **AIDS patients.**

. . . .

CYTOMEGALOVIRUS (CMV) PNEUMONITIS

ID/CC	A **5-year-old** white male presents with malaise, anorexia, low-grade fever, sore throat of three days' duration, and dyspnea on exertion.
HPI	The child was raised abroad. His immunization status cannot be determined.
PE	VS: fever; tachycardia with occasional dropped beats. PE: **cervical lymphadenopathy** (= BULL'S-NECK APPEARANCE); smooth, **whitish-gray, adherent membrane over tonsils and pharynx;** no hepatosplenomegaly; diminished intensity of S1.
Labs	**Metachromatic granules** in **bacilli arranged in "Chinese character pattern"** on Albert stain of throat culture; *Corynebacterium diphtheriae* confirmed by growth observed on **Löffler's blood agar;** erythema and necrosis following intradermal injection of *C. diphtheriae* toxin (= POSITIVE SCHICK'S TEST); immunodiffusion studies (Elek's) confirm toxigenic strains of *C. diphtheriae*. ECG: ST-segment elevation; second-degree heart block.
Imaging	Echo: evidence of myocarditis.
Gross Pathology	Pharyngeal membranes not restricted to anatomic landmarks; pale and enlarged heart.
Micro Pathology	Polymorphonuclear exudate with bacteria; precipitated fibrin and cell debris forming membrane; marked hyperemia, edema, and necrosis of upper respiratory tract mucosa; exotoxin-induced myofibrillar hyaline degeneration; lysis of myelin sheath.
Treatment	Begin treatment on presumptive diagnosis pending lab results; specific antitoxin and penicillin or erythromycin; confirm eradication by repeat throat culture.
Discussion	A bacterial infection of the throat with systemic symptoms caused by a toxin, it is preventable by vaccine and produced by toxigenic *Corynebacterium diphtheriae,* a club-shaped, gram-positive aerobic bacillus. A **heat-labile exotoxin produces myocarditis and neuritis.** Diphtheria toxin is produced by beta-prophage-infected corynebacteria; it blocks EF-2 via ADP ribosylation and hence ribosomal function in protein synthesis. **FIRST AID** p.182

C. diptheria   GRR
exotoxin — myocarditis + neuritis
        EF 2

· ·

DIPHTHERIA

ID/CC	A 56-year-old male professor of veterinary medicine from **New Zealand** experiences sudden **high fever** with chills, **jaundice,** and **right upper quadrant pain** while attending a conference in the U.S.
HPI	His past history is unremarkable. He has been healthy and has been physically active working in the field with sheep and breeding **dogs.**
PE	VS: fever; hypotension (BP 90/50). PE: **hepatomegaly;** jaundiced sclera; on palpation of epigastrium and right hypochondrium, abdomen is tender with no rebound tenderness.
Labs	CBC: leukocytosis with neutrophilia; slight eosinophilia. Strongly positive **immunoblot test for antibodies to echinococcal antigens;** elevated direct bilirubin and alkaline phosphatase.
Imaging	CT/US-Abdomen: **multiple large septated liver cysts** impinging on bile ducts, producing biliary dilatation (due to obstruction).
Gross Pathology	Liver is most common site of invasion, but cysts may also form in lungs, kidney, bone, and brain; each cyst contains millions of scoleces and consists of two layers: an inner germinal layer and an outer laminated layer; usually surrounded by fibrotic reaction.
Micro Pathology	Giant cell reaction surrounding cyst with eosinophilic infiltration.
Treatment	Surgically remove cysts if possible; albendazole may be effective.
Discussion	A zoonosis produced by *Echinococcus granulosus;* acquired through the ingestion of food or drink contaminated with the feces of dogs or other carnivores that have eaten contaminated meat; humans are the intermediate host of parasitic larvae. Accidental spilling of cyst fluid, either spontaneously or during surgery, may result in secondary seeding or anaphylaxis and even death. Also known as **hydatid disease.**

. . . .

ECHINOCOCCOSIS

ID/CC   A 36-year-old woman with AIDS and fulminant **gram-negative** pneumonia develops a spiking **fever, chills,** and **delirium.**

HPI   She had been on a regimen of antibiotics for treatment of her pneumonia, but her symptoms failed to resolve.

PE   VS: severe **hypotension; tachycardia; tachypnea.** PE: pallor; extremities warm (vs. other forms of shock); cyanosis; flattened JVP; patient confused and uncooperative; no focal neurologic signs; funduscopic exam normal; no meningeal signs.

Labs   CBC: **leukocytosis** with left-shift neutrophilia; band forms increased. UA: oliguria; abundant WBCs but no casts. *E. coli* on urine and blood culture. ABGs: hypoxia; hypercarbia (metabolic acidosis).

Imaging   CXR-PA: noncardiogenic pulmonary edema suggestive of **acute respiratory distress syndrome (ARDS).**

Gross Pathology   Bacterial endotoxins lead to a severe decrease in systemic vascular resistance, leading to vascular collapse; can lead rapidly to ARDS, acute tubular necrosis, disseminated intravascular coagulation (DIC), multiple organ failure, or death.

Micro Pathology   N/A

Treatment   Fluid resuscitation with monitoring of all cardiovascular parameters; IV antibiotics (initially broad spectrum, then dictated by culture sensitivity); management of ARDS with oxygen and positive end-expiratory pressure.

Discussion   Septic or endotoxic shock usually results from infection by microorganisms that trigger the release of mediators which act as vasodilators and myocardial depressants. Gram-negative bacteria release endotoxins whereas gram-positive bacteria release exotoxins. **FIRST AID** p.177

lipid A

. . . .

ENDOTOXIC SHOCK

ID/CC	A 28-year-old Guatemalan male is brought to the hospital complaining of **severe headache** and fever over the past two weeks.
HPI	As a political dissident, he spent four months in a **refugee camp** in southern Mexico before entering the U.S.
PE	VS: fever (40 C). PE: papilledema and delirium; bilateral swelling of parotid glands one week later; toxic facies; maculopapular **rash** on trunk and extremities; **face, palms, and soles spared**; mild splenomegaly.
Labs	**Positive Weil–Felix reaction** to OX-19 strains of *Proteus*; rise in complement fixation titer for *R. prowazekii*; specific antibodies. UA: proteinuria; microscopic hematuria.
Imaging	N/A
Gross Pathology	Myocarditis and pneumonia may be present; cerebral edema central to peripheral spreading maculopapular rash.
Micro Pathology	**Zenker's degeneration of striated muscle;** thrombosis and endothelial proliferation of capillaries with abundant rickettsiae and perivascular cuffing; accumulation of lymphocytes; microglia and macrophages (**typhus nodules**) in brain.
Treatment	Tetracycline; chloramphenicol.
Discussion	A febrile illness caused by *Rickettsia prowazekii,* a gram-negative, nonmotile, obligate intracellular parasite; transmitted via body lice and associated with war, famine, and crowded living conditions. The rash should be differentiated from Rocky Mountain spotted fever, which starts peripherally on the wrists and ankles and also includes the palms and soles.

obligate intracell.
Rickettsia
Chlamydia   tetracyc.
treats
facultative intracell
Mycobacteria
brucella
francisella
Listeria
gonorrhea

· ·

EPIDEMIC TYPHUS (RICKETTSIA PROWAZEKII)

ID/CC	A 4-year-old male presents with **fever, hoarseness,** and respiratory distress because of partial **airway obstruction.**
HPI	The child is also **unable to speak clearly and has pain while swallowing** (= ODYNOPHAGIA).
PE	VS: fever; tachypnea. PE: **patient is leaning forward with neck hyperextended and chin protruding; drooling;** marked suprasternal and infrasternal retraction of chest; **inspiratory stridor** on auscultation.
Labs	Culture of throat swab (no role in management of acute disease) reveals penicillinase-resistant *H. influenzae*; blood cultures also positive.
Imaging	XR-Neck: marked edema of epiglottis and aryepiglottic folds (= "THUMBS-UP" SIGN).
Gross Pathology	Epiglottis is cherry-red, swollen, and "angry-looking." Rapid cellulitis of epiglottis and surrounding tissue leads to progressive blockage of airway.
Micro Pathology	N/A
Treatment	Preservation of airway; IV cefuroxime.
Discussion	The principal cause of acute epiglottitis in children and adults is *H. influenzae* type b; *S. aureus* and *S. pneumoniae* can also cause epiglottitis in adults. Characterized by rapid onset. **FIRST AID** p.183

· ·

EPIGLOTTITIS (H. INFLUENZAE)

ID/CC	A 4-year-old female is brought to the pediatrician because of **lack of appetite**; nausea and **vomiting; chronic, foul-smelling diarrhea;** and a **bloated** sensation.
HPI	She has been in several **day-care centers** over the past three years.
PE	**Low weight and height** for age; mild epigastric tenderness.
Labs	**Binucleate, pear-shaped, flagellated trophozoites** (= *GIARDIA LAMBLIA*) on freshly passed stool; cysts found on stool exam.
Imaging	N/A
Gross Pathology	N/A
Micro Pathology	N/A
Treatment	Metronidazole.
Discussion	The most **common protozoal infection in children in the U.S.,** it is transmitted mainly through **contaminated food or water** and causes malabsorption.

. . . .

GIARDIASIS

ID/CC	A 21-year-old female college student complains of low-grade fever along with **pain** and **swelling** in the left knee of five days' duration.
HPI	She had been to her family physician two weeks ago because of **dysuria** and a **purulent vaginal discharge** (due to gonococcal infection) and was given an "antibiotic shot." She was asymptomatic until four days ago. She then developed **fever, chills,** and pain in both wrists and in her left ankle, which disappeared when the pain appeared in her left knee (= MIGRATORY POLYARTHRALGIA).
PE	Swollen, tender, warm left knee with **limited range of motion**; white vaginal discharge.
Labs	Intracellular, bean-shaped gram-negative diplococci (= GONOCOCCI) and **markedly elevated WBC count** on urethral smear and **synovial fluid aspirate.**
Imaging	XR-Knee: soft tissue swelling.
Gross Pathology	N/A
Micro Pathology	N/A
Treatment	**IV ceftriaxone.**
Discussion	Almost always accompanied by synovitis and effusion, gonococcal arthritis can rapidly destroy articular cartilage and is often associated with skin rash and C5, C6, and C7 complement deficiencies. Single joints are usually affected, most often the hip > shoulder > elbow > wrist > sternoclavicular joint.

GONOCOCCAL ARTHRITIS

ID/CC	A 19-year-old white male presents with **burning urination; profuse, greenish-yellow, purulent urethral discharge;** staining of his underwear; and urethral pain.
HPI	Four days ago, he had **unprotected sexual contact** with a prostitute.
PE	**Mucopurulent** and slightly blood-tinged urethral discharge; normal testes and epididymis; no urinary retention.
Labs	Smear of urethral discharge reveals **intracellular gram-negative diplococci** in WBCs; gonococcal infection confirmed by inoculation into **Thayer–Martin medium.**
Imaging	N/A
Gross Pathology	Abundant, purulent urethral exudate.
Micro Pathology	N/A
Treatment	Ceftriaxone plus doxycycline or erythromycin for **possible coinfection with *Chlamydia*.**
Discussion	A common STD caused by *Neisseria gonorrhoeae*, it may involve the throat, anus, rectum, epididymis, cervix, fallopian tubes, prostate, and joints; conjunctivitis is also found in neonates.

metabolizes glucose only
N. mening. → glu + maltose

ID/CC	A 25-year-old homosexual male visits a health clinic complaining of headache, low-grade fever, and a **painful skin rash in the perianal area.**
HPI	He has no history of penile ulcerations and admits to **unprotected anal sex** with **multiple partners.**
PE	Perianal **vesicular** rash in clusters **on erythematous base;** no penile ulceration; painful inguinal lymphadenopathy.
Labs	**Multinucleated giant cells with intranuclear inclusions** surrounded by clear halo on Pap-stained section of scrapings from base of vesicles.
Imaging	N/A
Gross Pathology	Clear liquid in vesicles; secondary bacterial infection may result; painful ulcerations when vesicles rupture.
Micro Pathology	Inflammatory infiltrate with abundant lymphocytes.
Treatment	**Acyclovir.**
Discussion	An enveloped, double-stranded DNA virus transmitted by sexual contact, it has a **tendency to recur** and can be **transmitted to the fetus through the birth canal.** **FIRST AID** p.201

HERPES SIMPLEX (TYPE 2)

ID/CC	A 27-year-old white female complains of **mouth ulcers, prolonged fever,** flulike symptoms, and increasing fatigue and weight loss over the past two months.
HPI	She recently moved from a large metropolitan area to a farm in **Ohio,** where she spent one week cleaning a **pigeons' loft.**
PE	VS: fever (38.5 C). PE: pallor; weight loss; enlarged liver and spleen; generalized lymphadenopathy; scattered, sibilant rales over lung fields.
Labs	CBC/PBS: anemia; leukopenia. Small, budding fungus found **intracellularly in reticuloendothelial cells** (macrophages) on silver stain; elevated LDH; positive blood culture for dimorphic fungus.
Imaging	CXR: nonsegmental shifting pneumonic infiltrates; mediastinal adenopathy with popcorn calcifications; bilateral **hilar adenopathy.** CT-Abdomen: splenic calcifications.
Gross Pathology	Nodules with granuloma formation; central area of necrosis and caseation with sclerosis and calcification; any organ may be involved, mainly reticuloendothelial system (RES) and adrenals.
Micro Pathology	**Granulomas** with epithelioid cells, Langhans' giant cells, and organisms within macrophages; in disseminated disease, organisms present in RES throughout body with proliferation.
Treatment	Itraconazole; amphotericin B.
Discussion	A systemic fungal infection sometimes resembling TB that is caused by *Histoplasma capsulatum,* a dimorphic fungus. The yeast form is found intracellularly; the mold form is found in soil associated with **bird or bat feces.** Transmitted by inhalation of mold spores, it varies in intensity from asymptomatic to fulminant (in immunocompromised patients).

. . . .

HISTOPLASMOSIS

ID/CC	A 38-year-old white female visits her gynecologist for a **routine Pap smear.**
HPI	She admits to early sexual activity, **many sexual partners, and unprotected sex.**
PE	Pallor; cervical tenderness; a few small, raised, flat lesions on cervix; **genital warts** also seen on vulva (= CONDYLOMATA ACUMINATA).
Labs	Presence of HPV in cervical cells revealed on **DNA hybridization and immunofluorescent antibody assays** for viral antigen.
Imaging	N/A
Gross Pathology	N/A
Micro Pathology	Rounded basophilic cells on Pap smear with **large nuclei** occupying most of surface; **nuclei show mitoses and coarse clumping of chromatin with perinuclear halo** (= SEVERE KOILOCYTIC DYSPLASIA).
Treatment	Conization or local excision with follow-up.
Discussion	Infection with **HPV types 16, 18, and 31** is strongly associated with **cervical cancer** preceded by dysplasia.

. . . .

HUMAN PAPILLOMAVIRUS (HPV)

ID/CC	A 57-year-old **black** male complains to his doctor of increasing weakness, **swollen glands in the armpits and groin,** and a feeling of **heaviness in the abdomen** (due to hepatosplenomegaly).
HPI	The patient is an immigrant from **Trinidad and Tobago** and has a history of nonresolving skin rashes and recurrent respiratory infections.
PE	Marked **pallor;** extensive papular skin rash with few erythematous plaques over abdomen; **generalized lymphadenopathy and hepatosplenomegaly.**
Labs	CBC/PBS: marked **leukocytosis (83,000)** with relative **lymphocytosis** and **atypical lymphocytes. Increased LDH; hypercalcemia.**
Imaging	CXR: normal.
Gross Pathology	N/A
Micro Pathology	Skin biopsy reveals infiltration by **leukemic CD4+ T lymphocytes.**
Treatment	Aggressive combination chemotherapy.
Discussion	Adult T-cell leukemia/lymphoma (ATLL) is associated with HTLV-1 type C, a retrovirus that has a higher incidence in **blacks** from the **Caribbean and southeastern U.S.** as well as in people from **southern Japan and sub-Saharan Africa.**

. . . .

HUMAN T-CELL LEUKEMIA VIRUS TYPE 1 (HTLV-1)

ID/CC	A 20-year-old male college student complains of **sore throat, fever, swollen lymph nodes on the back of his neck,** anorexia, cough, and **malaise** of 10 days' duration.
HPI	He was initially given **ampicillin** by his school nurse, after which he developed an extensive **skin rash.**
PE	VS: fever. PE: enlargement of submaxillary and **cervical lymph nodes; exudative tonsillitis;** petechiae on soft palate; slightly **enlarged spleen and liver.**
Labs	CBC/PBS: anemia; thrombocytopenia; leukocytosis with absolute **lymphocytosis (50%); atypical lymphocytes.** Elevated ALT, AST, and bilirubin; **positive heterophil antibody test** (= PAUL–BUNNELL TEST); IgM antibodies to viral capsid antigen/monospot positive.
Imaging	N/A
Gross Pathology	Enlarged spleen, lymph nodes, and, to lesser extent, liver; hepatitis may be present along with brain involvement; splenic rupture rare complication.
Micro Pathology	Proliferation of reticuloendothelial system; infiltration of spleen by atypical lymphocytes.
Treatment	**Supportive;** treat secondary strep infection accordingly.
Discussion	A systemic viral infection caused by Epstein–Barr virus (EBV), a herpesvirus, it is transmitted through respiratory droplets and saliva. In developed countries, it most commonly affects teenagers and young adults ("kissing disease"); in underdeveloped countries, it is seen as a subclinical infection of early childhood. EBV infection is associated with an increased risk of **Burkitt's lymphoma** and **nasopharyngeal carcinoma.** FIRST AID p.201

INFECTIOUS MONONUCLEOSIS (EBV)

ID/CC   A 40-year-old male smoker complains of acute-onset **high fever,** chills, a **nonproductive cough,** tachypnea, and **pleuritic chest pain.**

HPI   A number of **similar cases** have been reported in his workplace in recent months. The patient admits to significant alcohol and tobacco consumption and uses a **humidifier** at night.

PE   VS: fever; dyspnea. PE: rales present bilaterally on auscultation.

Labs   Sputum exam with Gram stain reveals no pathogenic organisms. CBC: neutrophilic leukocytosis. Cold agglutinins absent; indirect fluorescent antibody technique reveals stable titer of > 1:256 (considered diagnostic); **direct immunofluorescent** staining of sputum confirms presence of *Legionella.*

Imaging   CXR-PA: bilateral diffuse, patchy infiltrates and **ill-defined nodules.**

Gross Pathology   Nodular areas of consolidation which may progress to involvement of one or more lobes of the lung.

Micro Pathology   Alveolar exudate with PMNs, macrophages, and fibrin; in more severe cases, destruction of alveolar septa.

Treatment   Erythromycin.

Discussion   Legionnaire's disease is caused by a filamentous, flagellated, aerobic gram-negative, motile bacillus, *Legionella pneumophila,* and is more common in immunocompromised patients. Epidemiologic studies have established **drinking water** and **air conditioners** as the sources of outbreak.
FIRST AID p.183

. . . .

LEGIONELLA PNEUMONIA (LEGIONNAIRE'S DISEASE)

ID/CC	A 30-year-old **Pakistani immigrant** complains of chronic **fever,** weight loss, increased abdominal girth, a feeling of heaviness, and appetite loss.
HPI	Almost one year ago, the patient had a small, pruritic red **papule** on his left arm that was caused by an insect bite and disappeared spontaneously.
PE	**Skin darkening;** trophic changes in hair; **massive** nontender, hard **splenomegaly;** hepatomegaly without jaundice; generalized lymphadenopathy; peripheral edema; ecchymosis.
Labs	CBC/PBS: **anemia, leukopenia, thrombocytopenia** (= PANCYTOPENIA) and monocytosis; **amastigotes in buffy coat.** Hypergammaglobulinemia; decreased albumin; increased ALT and AST.
Imaging	CT/US-Abdomen: splenomegaly.
Gross Pathology	**Massively enlarged spleen;** also greatly increased in weight, dark-colored, and congested with Leishman–Donovan bodies.
Micro Pathology	Proliferation of reticuloendothelial system cells; biopsy or aspiration reveals parasite-filled macrophages in infected locations.
Treatment	Pentavalent antimony (e.g., **sodium stibogluconate**); amphotericin B or pentamidine isethionate.
Discussion	Also known as kala azar, it is a zoonosis that is produced by *Leishmania donovani* and transmitted through the bite of the *Phlebotomus* sandfly. Associated with a high fatality rate when left untreated.

sandfly
parasite in MØ's
splenomegaly - feeling of heaviness
Donovan bodies

LEISHMANIASIS

ID/CC	A 26-year-old male from India presents with a **hypopigmented, anesthetic skin patch** over the left side of his face.
HPI	He also complains of an occasional "electric current"-like sensation radiating from his left elbow to his hand.
PE	Dry, hypopigmented, anesthetic patch over left cheek; left **ulnar nerve enlarged and palpable;** eye, ear, nose, and throat exam normal; testes normal (vs. signs that are often demonstrable in lepromatous leprosy).
Labs	Glucose-6-phosphate dehydrogenase (G6PD) levels within normal range (done to prevent dapsone-associated hemolysis); slit skin smears reveal few **acid-fast bacilli;** skin biopsy from patch diagnostic of tuberculoid leprosy.
Imaging	N/A
Gross Pathology	**Single or small number of lesions** with macular or raised edges.
Micro Pathology	Skin biopsy reveals many well-formed epithelioid granulomas with very **few** acid-fast bacilli.
Treatment	Chemotherapy with rifampin and dapsone.
Discussion	Caused by *Mycobacterium leprae*, an acid-fast bacillus. The organism has two unique properties: it is thermolabile, growing best at 27°C to 30°C, and it divides very slowly; generation time is 12–14 days. Consequently, leprosy in humans typically evolves very slowly. Tuberculoid leprosy predominantly affects the skin with limited nerve involvement (most commonly ulnar and peroneal); **lepromatous leprosy** has diffuse involvement of the skin, eyes, nerves, and upper airway with disfigurement of the hands and face (**leonine facies**).

. . . .

LEPROSY (TUBERCULOID)

ID/CC	A **2-week-old** female is brought to the emergency room because of **high fever and convulsions.**
HPI	She also has an **extensive skin rash** on her legs and trunk.
PE	VS: fever. PE: generalized hypotonia; **extensive maculopapular skin rash; nuchal rigidity; involuntary flexion of hips when flexing neck** (= BRUDZINSKI'S SIGN).
Labs	CBC: neutrophilic leukocytosis. LP: elevated CSF cell count (750 cells/mL), mostly **neutrophils;** elevated CSF protein; low CSF sugar. Gram-positive, facultative, intracellular, nonsporulating bacilli on Gram stain and culture.
Imaging	N/A
Gross Pathology	Purulent meningitis.
Micro Pathology	Bacillus provokes both acute suppurative reaction with neutrophilic infiltration and chronic granuloma formation with focal necrosis.
Treatment	IV antibiotics (high-dose ampicillin).
Discussion	Caused by *Listeria monocytogenes.* Bacterial infection may occur early (acquired **in utero**) or later (drinking **contaminated milk**) in neonatal life. May be rapidly fatal if disseminated. Also occurs in adults immune-compromised by disease (e.g., renal disease or HIV). *E. coli* and *S. agalactiae* are two other common causes of neonatal meningitis.

· ·

LISTERIOSIS

ID/CC	A 12-year-old male presents with **fatigue, fever,** headache, **fleeting joint pain,** and a **reddish rash** on his trunk and left leg of one week's duration.
HPI	The patient is a native of **Connecticut** and attended a summer camp in the state's national park two weeks ago. He recalls having noticed a **tick bite** on his leg about two weeks ago.
PE	VS: fever. PE: red macule on site of bite that has grown circumferentially; **active border and central clearing** (= ERYTHEMA CHRONICUM MIGRANS); femoral lymphadenopathy; mild neck stiffness; normal CNS exam.
Labs	Positive IgM ELISA for *Borrelia burgdorferi*; diagnosis confirmed by Western blot assay. ECG: normal. LP: lymphocytic pleocytosis; increased proteins. *Borrelia burgdorferi* grown on Noguchi medium.
Imaging	N/A
Gross Pathology	Erythema chronicum migrans (ECM) is characteristic of Lyme disease; must be minimum of 5 cm in diameter for diagnosis to be made; center may desquamate, ulcerate, or necrose; satellite lesions sometimes seen; may spontaneously disappear with time.
Micro Pathology	N/A
Treatment	Doxycycline; amoxicillin; ceftriaxone.
Discussion	The most common disease transmitted by vectors in the U.S., it is caused by *Borrelia burgdorferi*, a spirochete, and is transmitted through *Ixodes* species tick bites. Ticks acquire *Borrelia burgdorferi* from deer mice, which are the natural reservoir. There are three recognized stages: stage 1 consists of ECM and constitutional symptoms; stage 2, cardiac or neurologic involvement; and stage 3, persistent migratory arthritis, synovitis, and **atrophic patches on the distal extremities** (= ACRODERMATITIS CHRONICUM ATROPHICANS).

. . . .

LYME DISEASE

ID/CC	A 57-year-old black female from Kenya complains of increasing weight and **edema of the lower legs** with difficulty walking.
HPI	Over the years she has had episodes of **fever with swelling of inguinal lymph nodes** and itching. She has also had numerous attacks of malaria.
PE	Inguinal lymph nodes indurated and slightly increased in size; marked deformity in both legs with **thickening of skin** and greatly **increased diameter; rubbery consistency.**
Labs	PBS: several **microfilariae;** prominent **eosinophilia.**
Imaging	Lymphangiogram: partial lymphatic obstruction at iliac level.
Gross Pathology	Presence of adult worms in lymphatics; marked fibrosis surrounding obstructed vessels.
Micro Pathology	Granulomatous reaction with plasma cell and lymphocytic infiltration; giant cell formation; intense fibroblastic hyperplasia.
Treatment	**Diethylcarbamazine; ivermectin;** surgery in advanced cases.
Discussion	A chronic disease due to lymphatic obstruction caused by several types of filarial roundworms, mainly *Wuchereria bancrofti* and *Brugia malayi;* transmitted by **mosquito bites.** Also known as elephantiasis.

· ·

LYMPHATIC FILARIASIS

ID/CC	A 25-year-old male complains of swollen, **tender masses in his groin** and very painful **genital ulcers** of one week's duration.
HPI	The patient admits to having had **unprotected sex** with multiple partners.
PE	**Swollen,** erythematous, tender **inguinal nodes,** usually bilateral, with draining sinuses (= INGUINAL ADENITIS, BUBOES); multiple small genital lesions.
Labs	Inguinal node biopsy diagnostic; **positive complement fixation test; positive immunofluorescence test.**
Imaging	N/A
Gross Pathology	Primary lesion is ulcerated nodule; gives rise to **inguinal bubo,** an enlarged lymph node sometimes characterized by fistulous tract formation; balanitis, phimosis, and rectal involvement with stricture may also be present.
Micro Pathology	Neutrophilic infiltration of primary lesion with areas of necrosis; lymphoid hyperplasia of lymph nodes with foci of macrophage accumulation; abscess formation with fibrosis.
Treatment	**Doxycycline;** tetracycline azithromycin; erythromycin; SMX–TMP; ceftriaxone; ciprofloxacin.
Discussion	An STD due to *Chlamydia trachomatis* (L1, L2, L3). Counseling should be given about other STDs (e.g., AIDS, syphilis, gonorrhea).

. . . .

LYMPHOGRANULOMA VENEREUM

ID/CC   A 30-year-old missionary comes to the emergency room complaining of **high fever, chills, severe headache,** and confusion.

HPI   Upon returning from **Africa** two weeks ago, he began to feel weak and experienced backaches, pain behind the eyes, and sleepiness.

PE   VS: fever (39 C); tachycardia. PE: pallor; profuse **sweating;** mild splenomegaly without lymphadenopathy.

Labs   CBC/PBS: anemia; thrombocytopenia; **plasmodia in erythrocytes on thick peripheral blood smear.** Slight hyperbilirubinemia and hypoglycemia.

Imaging   N/A

Gross Pathology   Liver and spleen moderately enlarged and soft in consistency, with sequestration and hemolysis of erythrocytes and macrophages; hyperplasia of Kupffer cells; malarial pigment in spleen and liver; brain capillaries may show thromboses.

Micro Pathology   Hypertrophy of phagocytic system; ischemic necrosis surrounding occluded blood vessels in brain.

Treatment   Chloroquine; quinine for cerebral malaria; sulfadiazine–pyrimethamine, mefloquine, tetracycline for areas with chloroquine-resistant strains; primaquine for radical treatment.

Cinchonism: tinnitus, arrythmyas

Discussion   Transmitted by female *Anopheles* mosquitoes. *Plasmodium falciparum* may be lethal, producing cerebral malaria. Other types include *P. vivax, P. ovale,* and *P. malariae.*
FIRST AID p.193

MALARIA

ID/CC	A **3-year-old** female is brought to the emergency room with a **high fever of seven days' duration,** accompanied by **redness of the eyes,** persistent dry **cough,** and **coryza.**
HPI	Her family doctor had treated her illness as a viral URI, but no improvement was seen. One day before her admission, her mother noticed a **skin rash starting behind her ears and face** that has now spread to her trunk and extremities.
PE	Pallor; injected conjunctiva; hyperemic throat; erythematous maculopapular rash on face, neck, trunk, and extremities; retroauricular lymphadenopathy; **bluish-gray spots surrounded by erythematous areola on buccal mucosa in region of first molar** (= KOPLIK'S SPOTS).
Labs	CBC: **leukopenia.**
Imaging	N/A
Gross Pathology	**Koplik's spots** pathognomonic of measles; appearance presages rash by approximately two days; uniform lesions (vs. varicella).
Micro Pathology	Lymphocytic dermal infiltration; multinucleated giant cells in reticuloendothelial system (= WARTHIN–FINKELDEY CELLS).
Treatment	No specific antiviral therapy available; treat complications.
Discussion	Also called **rubeola;** not to be confused with rubella. Measles is produced by a **paramyxovirus** and is transmitted by **respiratory droplets;** a vaccine is available. Measles has an incubation period of 10–14 days. Sequelae include encephalitis, subacute sclerosing panencephalitis (SSPE), and giant cell pneumonia. **FIRST AID** p.200

rubeolla = measles
Koplik spots
Warthin - Finkeldey giant cells
SSPE

ID/CC	A 12-year-old white female is brought to the emergency room because of sudden **fever** with **chills, severe headache,** pain in the extremities and back, **stiff neck,** and generalized rash; she also **fainted** while in school.
HPI	She had been well until admission, with no relevant history. In the emergency room, she **vomits bright red blood** twice.
PE	VS: tachycardia; hypotension (BP 70/50). PE: altered sensorium; pallor; moist, cold skin; nuchal rigidity and positive Kernig's sign; **petechial rash** all over body; minimal papilledema on funduscopic exam; no focal neurologic signs.
Labs	**Hypoglycemia.** Lytes: **hyponatremia; hyperkalemia.** CBC/PBS: thrombocytopenia; **neutrophilic leukocytosis.** LP: **CSF** cloudy and under increased pressure; increased proteins; low sugar. **Gram-negative diplococci** (*Neisseria meningitidis*) **seen within and outside WBCs** on Gram stain. Negative India ink and ZN stain; growth of meningococci later revealed on blood culture.
Imaging	CT-Head: normal. CT-Abdomen: bilateral adrenal hemorrhage. → Watehouse - Friedrichson
Gross Pathology	**Bilateral adrenal hemorrhagic necrosis;** skin necrosis; pyogenic meningitis.
Micro Pathology	Meningeal hyperemia with abundant purulent exudate; diplococcus-containing PMNs; acute hemorrhagic necrosis of adrenal glands.
Treatment	Steroid replacement; IV fluids; dopamine; IV penicillin G; prophylactic rifampin for close contacts.
Discussion	A **fulminant disease** caused by several groups of *Neisseria meningitidis*; the cause of death is adrenal necrosis with vascular collapse. A meningococcal vaccine is available. Also known as **Waterhouse–Friedrichsen's syndrome.**

. . . .

MENINGOCOCCEMIA

ID/CC A 24-year-old white female with **insulin-dependent diabetes mellitus (IDDM)** is hospitalized for **ketoacidosis** following a night out drinking; on the fifth day she develops right **periorbital swelling** and mucopurulent postnasal discharge that **fails to respond to antibiotics.**

HPI She admits to irregular adherence to glucose control and insulin dosing.

PE Right **periorbital** and paranasal **edema;** swelling of conjunctiva (= CHEMOSIS); exophthalmos; **black ulceration of nasal mucosa; third cranial nerve (CN III) palsy.**

Labs **Large, irregular, nonseptate hyphae branching at wide (> 90°) angles** on nasal culture.

aspergillus is 45°

Imaging XR-Plain: opacification of paranasal sinuses.

Gross Pathology Necrotic destruction of paranasal sinuses and orbit with dissemination to lung and brain.

Micro Pathology Purulent arteritis with thrombi composed of hyphae; inflammation and necrosis with polymorphonuclear infiltrate.

Treatment Maintain tighter glucose control; amphotericin B; surgical drainage.

Discussion A phycomycosis produced by _Mucor_ and _Rhizopus_ molds, it should be suspected in cases of antibiotic-resistant sinusitis, especially in the presence of underlying diabetes, lymphoma, or leukemia. **FIRST AID** p.189

. . . .

MUCORMYCOSIS 90°

ID/CC	A **6-year-old** white male presents with fever, nausea, vomiting, **swelling,** and tenderness of the **mandibular angle**; he finds it difficult to talk, eat, or swallow.
HPI	Two of his classmates were diagnosed with mumps two weeks ago. There is no vaccination record.
PE	VS: fever. PE: outward and upward displacement of ear; **obliterated mandibular hollow; orifice of Stensen's duct swollen and hyperemic; right testicle enlarged and painful.**
Labs	CBC: leukopenia with **lymphocytosis. Hyperamylasemia;** positive complement fixation antibodies.
Imaging	N/A
Gross Pathology	Parotid glands enlarged with areas of necrosis and mononuclear infiltrate; encephalitis, orchitis, oophoritis, meningitis, and pancreatitis may also be present.
Micro Pathology	Examination of parotid glands reveals perivascular mononuclear, lymphocytic, and plasma cell infiltrate with necrosis; ductal obstruction and edema; testicular interstitial edema; perivascular cerebral lymphocytic cuffing.
Treatment	Supportive; analgesics for pain; treat complications.
Discussion	A systemic infection caused by the mumps virus, an RNA paramyxovirus, it is transmitted by droplets and direct contact. Bilateral testicular involvement may lead to sterility; one of the most common causes of pancreatitis in children. A vaccine is available with measles and rubella (MMR).

mumps + measles (rubeola) are paramyxo

ID/CC	A 20-year-old male college student presents with a **productive cough,** headache, **malaise,** runny nose, and **fever.**
HPI	He has a history of sore throat preceding the onset of the **cough, which initially was nonproductive.**
PE	VS: fever. PE: mild respiratory distress; auscultation reveals fine to medium rales over right lower lobe.
Labs	Gram stain of sputum negative; routine cultures of both blood and sputum negative. CBC: **leukocyte count normal.** Fourfold rise in complement fixation titer in paired sera; **cold agglutinin titer > 1:128.**
Imaging	CXR: patchy alveolar infiltrates involving right lower lobe; appears worse than the clinical picture.
Gross Pathology	Unilateral lower lobe pneumonia with firm, red pulmonary parenchyma in affected areas.
Micro Pathology	Bronchial mucosa congested and edematous; inflammatory response consists of perivascular lymphocytes initially and PMNs later in infection. **Organism lacks cell wall** (thus penicillins and cephalosporins are ineffective).
Treatment	Erythromycin.
Discussion	Mycoplasma pneumonia is the **most common cause of primary atypical pneumonia.** Transmission is by droplet spread; rapidly infects those living in close quarters. **FIRST AID** p.188

. . . .

MYCOPLASMA PNEUMONIA

ID/CC	A 45-year-old white male undergoing **chemotherapy** for Hodgkin's lymphoma is brought to the emergency room by his wife because of shortness of breath and cyanosis.
HPI	For the past **three months,** he has been complaining of intermittent weakness, fever with chills, and foul-smelling, thick **greenish sputum.**
PE	VS: fever (38 C); tachypnea; tachycardia. PE: pallor; mild cyanosis; localized dullness with bronchial breathing; diminished breath sounds over left lower lobe.
Labs	CBC: leukocytosis with neutrophilia; anemia. Sputum culture reveals **gram-positive, filamentous, partially acid-fast** staining bacteria (due to *Nocardia*).
Imaging	CXR: nodular infiltrate in left lower lobe with air-fluid level (abscess) and left pleural effusion.
Gross Pathology	Lung lesions or disseminated lesions (brain, liver, kidney, subcutaneous tissue) consist of necrotic centers within regions of consolidation and abscess formation resembling pyogenic pneumonia.
Micro Pathology	Consolidation of alveoli with pus formation (exudate of PMNs and fibrin) and surrounding granulomatous reaction.
Treatment	Six-month course of SMX–TMP; surgery.
Discussion	A chronic bacterial infection seen in diabetics, leukemia and lymphoma patients, and **immunocompromised patients,** it usually involves the lungs with possible dissemination to the brain, subcutaneous tissue, and other organs. Caused by *Nocardia asteroides,* a branching, aerobic, gram-positive organism that is weakly acid fast; sometimes confused with *Mycobacterium tuberculosis.* **FIRST AID** p.183

Actinomyces in anaerobe

NOCARDIOSIS

ID/CC	A 56-year-old white female is referred to an ophthalmologist for an evaluation of **diminished visual acuity.**
HPI	She has spent most of her adult life as a missionary in rural **Senegal** and **Mali.** She admits to chronic **generalized itching, mostly while showering.**
PE	Wrinkling and loss of elastic tissue in skin; **marked hypopigmentation of shins;** 2- to 3-cm, nonfixed, firm, nontender subcutaneous **nodules on iliac bones, knees, and elbows;** chronic conjunctivitis, **sclerosing keratitis, chorioretinal lesions** on eye exam.
Labs	CBC/PBS: **eosinophilia.** Fifty-milligram dose of **diethylcarbamazine produces severe pruritus, rash, fever, and conjunctivitis** (= POSITIVE MAZZOTTI REACTION).
Imaging	N/A
Gross Pathology	N/A
Micro Pathology	Skin biopsy at iliac crest shows microfilariae.
Treatment	Ivermectin; suramin.
Discussion	Caused by *Onchocerca volvulus* and transmitted by the blackfly (= *SIMULIUM*), which breeds near rivers; hence it is also known as **"river blindness."** Larvae migrate through subcutaneous tissue, producing **painless soft tissue edema** (= CALABAR EDEMA); with time, subcutaneous nodules form and filariae obstruct dermal lymphatics, producing atrophy and hypopigmentation. Microfilariae concentrate in the eyes, leading to **chorioretinitis and blindness.**

· ·

ONCHOCERCIASIS

ID/CC	A 4-year-old white male presents with fever, chills, malaise, **pain,** and **immobility of the right knee** of one week's duration.
HPI	Two weeks ago the child fell while playing, but no abnormality was found by the school nurse.
PE	Overlying skin **warm and red; swelling** of distal third of thigh and knee; **tenderness** on palpation.
Labs	CBC: leukocytosis. **Elevated ESR.** Gram stain and culture confirm diagnosis and isolate pathogen.
Imaging	XR-Plain: early findings include soft tissue edema and thin line running parallel to diaphysis (**periosteal thickening**); later findings include bone erosion, subperiosteal abscess with periostitis, and sequestrum formation (due to detached necrotic cortical bone); involucrum formation (laminated periosteal reaction). MR: marrow edema; abscess. Indium-Labeled WBC-Scan: hot spot.
Gross Pathology	**New osteoblastic periosteal bone formation** (= INVOLUCRUM); **trapping of detached necrotic bone by involucrum** (= SEQUESTRUM); isolated localized abscess (= BRODIE'S ABSCESS); sinus tract formation, draining pus to skin.
Micro Pathology	Purulent exudate formation, usually metaphyseal, with ischemic necrosis of bone due to increased pressure of pus in rigid bone walls; vascular thrombosis.
Treatment	IV antibiotics according to sensitivity; **surgical debridement.**
Discussion	An acute pyogenic bone infection which, if left untreated, produces functional incapacity and deformities. The most common pathogen is *S. aureus;* less frequently *Streptococcus* and enterobacteria are involved. In sickle cell anemia *E. coli* and *Salmonella* species are seen; diabetics are at risk for *Pseudomonas* infection. Immunocompromised patients may show *Sporothrix schenckii* osteomyelitis; human bites, anaerobes; puncture wounds, *Pseudomonas aeruginosa;* and cat-bite wounds, *Pasteurella multocida.* **FIRST AID** p.190

. . . .

OSTEOMYELITIS

ID/CC   An 18-month-old white female presents with **irritability** together with bilateral, profuse, and foul-smelling **ear discharge** of two months' duration.

HPI   The patient had **recurrent URIs** last year, but her mother did not administer the complete course of antibiotics. The patient's mother has a history of feeding her child while lying down.

PE   Bilateral greenish-white ear discharge; **perforated tympanic membranes** in anteroinferior quadrant of both ears; **diminished mobility of tympanic membrane** on pneumatic otoscopy; on otoscopic exam, tympanic membrane found to be red, opaque, and bulging with loss of cone of light.

Labs   Gram-negative coccobacilli on Gram stain of discharge from tympanocentesis; *H. influenzae* seen on culture.

Imaging   N/A

Gross Pathology   Possible complications include **ingrowth of squamous epithelium on upper middle ear** (= CHOLESTEATOMA) if long-standing; conductive hearing loss; mastoiditis; brain abscess.

Micro Pathology   Hyperemia and edema of inner ear and throat mucosa; hyperemia of tympanic membrane; deposition of cholesterol crystals in keratinized epidermoid cells in cholesteatoma.

Treatment   Keep ear dry; <u>amoxicillin–clavulanic acid</u>; surgical drainage for severe otalgia; myringoplasty.

Discussion   The most common pediatric bacterial infection, it is caused by *E. coli, S. aureus, and Klebsiella pneumoniae* in neonates; in older children it is usually caused by pneumococcus *(S. pneumoniae)*, *H. influenzae, Moraxella catarrhalis,* and group A streptococcus. Resistant strains are becoming increasingly common.

ID/CC	A 12-year-old girl arrives in the emergency room with **pain, swelling, and limited motion** of her left hand; she also complains of fever and chills.
HPI	The girl was **bitten by a cat** three days ago while playing at a friend's house.
PE	Hand is erythematous, **shiny,** and **markedly edematous;** on palpation, hand is **tender** with fluctuation (cellulitis); limited passive and active motion; yellowish-green **purulent fluid** drains from wound; left epitrochlear and axillary **lymphadenitis** without lymphangitis.
Labs	**Gram-negative rods with bipolar staining** of abscess aspirate; **catalase and oxidase positive** (*Pasteurella multocida*).
Imaging	XR-Plain: soft tissue swelling; no periostitis or erosions (vs. osteomyelitis).
Gross Pathology	N/A
Micro Pathology	N/A
Treatment	**Incision and drainage, amoxicillin/clavulanate;** tetracycline; penicillin.
Discussion	*Pasteurella multocida* is the most common bacterium isolated from cat bite wounds and may progress to **osteomyelitis.** Human bite infections are most commonly caused by *Eikenella corrodens* and are treated with penicillin.

ID/CC	A 44-year-old male archaeologist presents with **high fever, malaise**, intense **headache, severe myalgia**, and **painful swelling in the inguinal region.**
HPI	He recently returned from a trip to **Arizona.**
PE	VS: tachycardia. PE: drowsy looking; no meningeal signs; pustule seen at site of an **insect bite** on left upper arm; **inguinal lymph nodes enlarged, fluctuant, and tender** (= BUBOES); no lesion on external genitalia.
Labs	CBC/PBS: normal; no malarial parasites. Gram-negative bacilli with **"safety pin"** appearance seen in aspirates from buboes; culture of aspirate reveals *Yersinia pestis.*
Imaging	N/A
Gross Pathology	Enlarged lymph nodes are necrotic and suppurative; pneumonic form shows lobar consolidation.
Micro Pathology	Numerous organisms in suppurative and necrotic lymph tissue.
Treatment	Streptomycin; tetracycline.
Discussion	Infection is usually acquired after contact with <u>rodents and fleas</u> in endemic areas (southwestern United States). Death rapidly ensues in the absence of treatment.

PLAGUE

ID/CC	An 11-year-old white male presents with a high-grade fever, a productive, **blood-tinged** cough, **mucoid sputum,** and **pleuritic left-sided chest pain** of a few days' duration.
HPI	The child had previously been well and is fully immunized.
PE	VS: fever; tachypnea. PE: use of accessory respiratory muscles; central trachea; decreased left respiratory excursion; **increased vocal fremitus in left infrascapular area with dullness to percussion; bronchial breathing** with coarse crackles heard over left lung area.
Labs	CBC: increased WBC count; preponderance of neutrophils. ABGs: hypoxemia without hypercapnia. **Gram-positive diplococci in sputum;** alpha-hemolytic colonies of gram-positive diplococci (*S. pneumoniae*) on blood agar culture.
Imaging	CXR: **homogenous opacification of left lower lobe** (= LOBAR CONSOLIDATION) with small left pleural effusion.
Gross Pathology	Consolidation of lung parenchyma passes through four stages: congestion and edema, red hepatization, gray hepatization, and resolution.
Micro Pathology	Vascular dilatation with hyperemia and alveolar edema; PMNs rich in purulent exudate; fibrin deposition; hardening of lung parenchyma with fibrin clotting inside alveoli (consolidation).
Treatment	Parenteral therapy with penicillin; monitor with radiologic imaging; supplemental oxygen for respiratory distress.
Discussion	*S. pneumoniae* is the most common cause of community-acquired pneumonia and produces typical lobar pneumonia.

. . . .

PNEUMOCOCCAL PNEUMONIA

ID/CC   A 32-year-old **HIV-positive male** presents with **progressively increasing dyspnea** over the past three weeks.

HPI   He also complains of a **dry**, painful **cough**, marked **fatigue**, and a continuous **low-grade fever**. He has been noncompliant with cotrimoxazole prophylaxis.

PE   VS: fever; marked **tachypnea**. PE: pallor; generalized lymphadenopathy; respiratory distress; **intercostal retraction**; mild central cyanosis; nasal flaring; coarse, crepitant rales auscultated at both lung bases.

Labs   ABGs: **hypoxemia out of proportion to clinical findings.** *Pneumocystis carinii* on **methenamine silver stain** of induced sputum or bronchoalveolar lavage; ELISA/Western blot positive for HIV. CBC: **leukopenia** with depressed CD4+ cell count. **Serum LDH typically elevated.**

Imaging   CXR: diffuse, bilaterally symmetrical **interstitial and alveolar infiltration** pattern, predominantly perihilar; no lymphadenopathy or effusion.

Gross Pathology   Congestion and consolidation of lungs with hypoaeration.

Micro Pathology   Eosinophilic exudate in alveoli with multiple 4- to 6-mm cysts containing oval bodies (= MEROZOITES) on lung biopsy or bronchial lavage; *Pneumocystis* abundant on Gomori methenamine silver stain.

Treatment   SMX–TMP; pentamidine; steroids for severe disease.

Discussion   An opportunistic infection that causes interstitial pneumonia in many **immunocompromised** patients. Traditionally it has been classified as a protozoan; however, *Pneumocystis carinii* ribosomal RNA indicates that the organism is **fungal**. Seen in the upper lobes in patients receiving inhaled pentamidine prophylaxis. Treat HIV patients prophylactically with SMX–TMP for *Pneumocystis carinii* pneumonia if the CD4 count is < 200. **FIRST AID** p.189

· ·

PNEUMOCYSTIS CARINII PNEUMONIA

ID/CC A 14-year-old male immigrant complains of malaise, **weight loss, fever, and night sweats** of six weeks' duration; he also has a mild cough that began to produce **bloody sputum** three days prior to his admission.

HPI The patient's **mother** has been diagnosed with pulmonary **tuberculosis** and is currently receiving treatment for it.

PE VS: mild fever. PE: **malnourished;** low height and weight for age; bronchial breath sounds with crepitant rales heard over right supramammary area.

Labs CBC/PBS: normocytic, normochromic anemia; WBC count normal with relative **lymphocytosis. Increased ESR;** sputum stained with ZN stain **positive for acid-fast bacilli;** positive radiometric culture for *Mycobacterium tuberculosis*; positive ELISA for TB; positive **intradermal tuberculin injection** (= MANTOUX TEST).

Imaging CXR: small cavity with streaky infiltrates in right upper lobe; hilar lymphadenopathy; calcified lung lesion (= GHON'S LESION); Ghon's lesion and calcified lymph node (= RANKE COMPLEX).

Gross Pathology **Primary tuberculosis** usually consists of **lesions in lower lung lobes** and in subpleural locations; cavitation rare; **secondary TB** or reinfection characterized by cavitary lesions usually located in **apical regions.**

Micro Pathology Multinucleated epithelioid **Langhans cells** surround core of **caseating necrosis** in lung parenchyma, producing fibroblastic reaction at periphery with lymphocytic infiltration and proliferation (= TUBERCLE).

Treatment Multiple drug therapy with isoniazid (INH), rifampin, ethambutol, pyrazinamide, and/or streptomycin.

Discussion Caused by *Mycobacterium tuberculosis,* an acid-fast, gram-positive aerobic bacillus. An **increasing incidence in AIDS patients** has been observed; drug resistance is becoming common. **FIRST AID** p.185

. . . .

PULMONARY TUBERCULOSIS

ID/CC   A 12-year-old white female is rushed to the emergency room because of **numbness** of the right foot and leg followed by **fever** and **convulsions**. The child **refuses to drink any fluids** (= HYDROPHOBIA).

HPI   She had been camping five weeks ago. When questioned, her mother recalls that one night the child had apparently stepped on **a bat that bit her in the right foot.**

PE   VS: no fever. PE: child is **disoriented, hyperventilating,** extremely agitated, and actively moving all four limbs; thus **difficult to restrain;** no meningeal signs; fundus normal; **saliva viscous and foaming.**

Labs   LP: lymphocytic pleocytosis with mildly elevated proteins and normal sugar in CSF. **Positive rabies antigen in corneal scrapings.**

Imaging   N/A

Gross Pathology   N/A

Micro Pathology   Characteristic **cytoplasmic inclusion bodies in Ammon's horn** (= NEGRI BODIES) (pathognomonic). hippocampus

Treatment   Supportive; almost always fatal; prevent with vaccine; postexposure prophylaxis with diploid cell vaccine and human immune globulin.

Discussion   A fatal viral disease transmitted to humans by the bites of **raccoons,** skunks, foxes, coyotes, dogs, cats, and bats. Rabies virus is an enveloped, single-stranded RNA virus. Rabies has a **long incubation period** (approximately 3–8 weeks); death usually results from respiratory failure. **FIRST AID** p.200

. . . .

RABIES

ID/CC   A 4-month-old girl brought in for a well-child visit is found to be **low in weight and height for her age** and to have **lens opacities** (due to congenital cataracts).

HPI   Her mother had a skin rash and fever during her **first trimester.** The mother states that when the child was born, she too had a **rash** like a "blueberry muffin" and was **jaundiced.**

PE   **Deaf** and **globally retarded;** malnourished; **microcephaly** and bulging anterior fontanelle; **microphthalmia** with unilateral left **cataract;** discrete black, patchy pigmentation found in retina on funduscopic exam; **hepatosplenomegaly;** **machinery murmur heard at second intercostal space** on left sternal border (due to **patent ductus arteriosus**).

Labs   CBC/PBS: leukopenia; thrombocytopenia. Increased serum bilirubin (both direct and indirect); rubella virus isolated from urine and saliva; markedly increased **IgM specific antibody for rubella.**

Imaging   XR-Plain: radiolucent (lytic) bone lesions (metaphyseal).

Gross Pathology   N/A

Micro Pathology   N/A

Treatment   None.

Discussion   Rubella infection is a transitory and unremarkable disease in children and adults, but if acquired **in utero it has devastating consequences.** It is vaccine preventable with measles-mumps-rubella (MMR) vaccine. Also known as German measles.

ID/CC	A 10-year-old female Asian immigrant presents with a **low-grade fever** and coryza of three days' duration.
HPI	She also complains of arthralgias and a **skin rash that began on her face and spread to her trunk.** Her mother says she cannot remember any details of her vaccination history.
PE	VS: fever. PE: maculopapular rash over face and trunk; **enlarged postauricular, posterior cervical, and occipital lymph nodes.**
Labs	CBC: leukopenia; thrombocytopenia. Rubella virus hemagglutination inhibition test demonstrates **fourfold rise in titer** to 1:32.
Imaging	N/A
Gross Pathology	Erythematous skin rash resembling rubeola measles but lighter in color and more discrete; similar distribution pattern in both.
Micro Pathology	N/A
Treatment	Symptomatic treatment.
Discussion	Caused by a togavirus; live attenuated rubella virus vaccine should be given to all infants and to susceptible girls before menarche. The course of illness is self-limiting and mild; the major complication is congenital rubella syndrome. Females with rubella can get **polyarthritis** secondary to immune complex deposition.

RUBELLA (GERMAN MEASLES)

ID/CC	A 10-year-old white female complains of difficulty swallowing, pain in both ears, and fever of one week's duration; she also complains of an extensive skin rash.
HPI	The child is fully immunized and has been well until now.
PE	VS: fever. PE: **extensive erythematous rash** (= "GOOSE-PIMPLE SUNBURN") on neck, groin, and axillae; desquamation and **peeling of fingertips;** circumoral pallor; **lines of hyperpigmentation with tiny petechiae** (= PASTIA'S SIGN) in antecubital fossae; **bright red lingual papillae superimposed on white coat** (= "STRAWBERRY TONGUE"); pharyngitis with exudative tonsillitis; cervical lymphadenopathy; normal eardrums.
Labs	CBC: leukocytosis with neutrophilia. **Group A beta-hemolytic** *Streptococcus pyogenes* on throat swab and culture; **elevated ASO titer.**
Imaging	N/A
Gross Pathology	Toxin-induced vasodilation; complications include otitis media, pneumonia, glomerulonephritis, osteomyelitis, and rheumatic fever.
Micro Pathology	Inflammatory polymorphonuclear epidermal infiltrate; interstitial nephritis; lymph node hyperplasia.
Treatment	Penicillin; erythromycin.
Discussion	A streptococcal infection characterized by morbilliform rash due to **hypersensitivity to erythrogenic toxin.**

. . . .

SCARLET FEVER

ID/CC	A 27-year-old Peace Corps volunteer working in the **Congo** is sent home after developing **fever, sweats, and abdominal pain** that have not responded to antimalarial treatment.
HPI	Five weeks ago, he developed **severe itching and a macular rash** (= SWIMMER'S ITCH) after swimming in a nearby pond.
PE	VS: fever. PE: moderate enlargement of liver and spleen; tender abdomen but no peritoneal irritation.
Labs	CBC/PBS: **marked eosinophilia.** Characteristic large parasite eggs with lateral spines may be found in stool specimen.
Imaging	Sigmoidoscopy: swollen and erythematous mucosa; many small ulcerations. CT/US-Abdomen: hepatosplenomegaly; portal vein dilatation.
Gross Pathology	Skin and liver sites of principal lesions in acute stage; eggs may be found in liver, lungs, intestines, pancreas, spleen, urogenital organs, and brain; chronic stage characterized by granuloma formation in bladder and liver (= PERIPORTAL FIBROSIS).
Micro Pathology	Granulomatous reaction and fibrosis.
Treatment	Praziquantel.
Discussion	Among the most common parasitic diseases in the world; infection is acquired by **swimming** in **snail-infested ponds** and lakes. Also known as bilharziasis. Long-standing infection may lead to portal hypertension.

SCHISTOSOMIASIS

ID/CC   A 36-year-old male executive comes to the emergency room because of the development of **sudden nausea, vomiting, and diarrhea** with **blood and mucus** (dysentery) as well as crampy abdominal pain for two days.

HPI   He had just returned from a business trip in **South America.**

PE   VS: low-grade fever. PE: mild dehydration; hyperactive bowel sounds; tender abdomen without definite peritoneal irritation.

Labs   **Leukocytes on stool examination;** *Shigella* isolated on stool culture; on microbiology, organism does not ferment lactose and is **not motile.**   Ln KEG

Imaging   N/A

Gross Pathology   N/A

Micro Pathology   *Shigella* enterotoxin acts by activating adenylate cyclase; organism invades intestinal mucosa.

Treatment   Rehydration with antibiotic therapy (ampicillin or SMX–TMP).

Discussion   Outbreaks occur primarily in areas with **overcrowding** and **poor hygiene** (fecal-oral transmission); **arthritis, conjunctivitis, and urethritis** (= REITER'S SYNDROME) may be complications in HLA-B27-positive individuals. Like *Salmonella, Shigella* causes bloody diarrhea by invading the intestinal mucosa, causing intestinal ulceration and inflammation. **FIRST AID** p.184

. . . .

SHIGELLOSIS

ID/CC   A 37-year-old **gardener** complains of lumps with **red streaks** on his arm and swelling of the axillary lymph nodes.

HPI   Two weeks ago, he **pricked his hand with a thorn** while pruning roses. A **nodule** then formed which subsequently **ulcerated** and filled with pus.

PE   Nonpainful nodular lesion on dorsum of hand with ulcer formation and suppuration; **tender, palpable inflammation and hardening of lymph vessels** (= LYMPHANGITIS); **swelling, inflammation, and suppuration of lymph nodes** (= LYMPHADENITIS); nonulcerated satellite nodules along course of lymphatics.

Labs   **Cigar-shaped budding cells** (= *SPOROTHRIX SCHENCKII*) visible in pus; diagnosis confirmed by culture of aspirate of nodule.

Imaging   N/A

Gross Pathology   **Nonpainful, soft, ulcerated nodule at inoculation site** (= SPOROTRICHOTIC CHANCRE); may extend to deep tissues and bone with osteitis and synovitis.

Micro Pathology   Usually area of suppuration with polymorphonuclear infiltrate surrounded by granulomatous reaction of varied intensity with epithelioid and giant cell formation; chlamydospore asteroid bodies present.

Treatment   Itraconazole; potassium iodide.

Discussion   Also called **"rose gardener's disease,"** it is a fungal infection caused by *Sporothrix schenckii,* a dimorphic fungus that lives on vegetation. It is typically transmitted by a thorn prick and causes localized infection with few systemic manifestations. **FIRST AID** p.189

. . . .

SPOROTRICHOSIS

ID/CC	A 9-year-old male complains of **pain during swallowing** (= ODYNOPHAGIA) for two days, accompanied by muscle aches, headache, and fever.
HPI	He has otherwise been in good health.
PE	VS: fever. PE: moderate erythema of pharynx; enlarged, **erythematous tonsils** covered with white **exudate**; tender cervical adenopathy.
Labs	CBC: neutrophilic leukocytosis. *Streptococcus pyogenes* isolated on throat swab and culture.
Imaging	N/A
Gross Pathology	Hyperemia and swelling of upper respiratory tract mucosa; cryptic enlargement of tonsils with purulent exudate; enlargement of regional lymph nodes.
Micro Pathology	Acute inflammatory response with polymorphonuclear infiltrate, hyperemia and edema with pus formation; hyperplasia of regional lymph nodes; dilatation of sinusoids.
Treatment	**Oral penicillin V.**
Discussion	An acute bacterial infection produced by gram-positive **cocci in chains** (*Streptococcus*); infections are more commonly caused by group A streptococcus. Complications due to immune-mediated cross-reactivity and molecular mimicking may include glomerulonephritis and rheumatic fever.

· ·

STREPTOCOCCAL PHARYNGITIS

ID/CC	A 7-year-old girl is seen by the embassy doctor in **Nigeria** for abdominal pain, **diarrhea, fever, dry cough,** and marked **dyspnea** of two weeks' duration.
HPI	She is the daughter of an American diplomat working in Nigeria. Despite her parent's admonitions, she frequently **walks barefoot.**
PE	VS: fever. PE: moderate respiratory distress; no cyanosis; no clubbing; coarse, crepitant rales and **wheezing** heard over both lung fields; mild abdominal tenderness.
Labs	CBC/PBS: **marked eosinophilia.** Typical **motile rhabditiform larvae** on sputum exam as well as in freshly passed stool; positive filarial complement fixation test.
Imaging	CXR: **bilateral, transient migratory infiltrates.**
Gross Pathology	Pneumonitis produced by migration of larvae through respiratory tract.
Micro Pathology	N/A
Treatment	**Thiabendazole;** ivermectin.
Discussion	Infestation is seen in the presence of **poor hygiene** and in tropical countries. Larvae penetrate the skin, gaining entrance to the venous system and to the lungs, and then ascend to enter the GI tract.

. . . .

STRONGYLOIDIASIS

ID/CC	A 54-year-old white female complains of **spiking fever, chills, loss of appetite,** several bouts of diarrhea, and **right upper quadrant pain.**
HPI	**Ten days ago** she underwent an apparently uncomplicated emergency **surgery for suppurative cholecystitis** and was subsequently discharged and sent home.
PE	VS: fever. PE: pallor; slight icterus; **pain on percussion of right costal region;** well-healed surgical wound with no evidence of infection; liver not palpable; crepitant rales on right lung base.
Labs	CBC: **elevated WBC count (17,000) with predominance of neutrophils.**
Imaging	CXR: elevated right hemidiaphragm; slight right pleural effusion. US/CT: **complex fluid collection below diaphragm.**
Gross Pathology	N/A
Micro Pathology	N/A
Treatment	Percutaneous drainage under ultrasonic or fluoroscopic guidance followed by regular blood and radiologic exams; surgical exploration and drainage.
Discussion	Most commonly occurs after abdominal surgery, mainly with septic, emergency procedures; typically presents one week or more postoperatively.

SUBDIAPHRAGMATIC ABSCESS

ID/CC	A 6-week-old male, the son of a **prostitute,** is brought to the family doctor because of persistent, sometimes **bloody mucopurulent nasal discharge, anal ulcers,** and a generalized **rash.**
HPI	The child was delivered at home, and the mother did not receive any prenatal care.
PE	Weak-looking, **icteric** infant with hoarse cry; does not move right limb (**pseudoparalysis**); bloody purulent discharge evident at nares; generalized lymphadenopathy; hepatosplenomegaly; **maculopapular rash** with desquamation on back and buttocks; **bullae on hands and feet.**
Labs	CBC: anemia. **VDRL** in both mother and child **positive;** direct hyperbilirubinemia; negative Coombs' test; *Treponema pallidum* seen on nasal exudate and anal ulcers.
Imaging	XR-Plain: periostitis of long bones; bilateral moth-eaten lesions; focal defect in proximal tibial epiphysis with increased density of epiphyseal line (= WIMBERGER'S SIGN).
Gross Pathology	Pathologic features seen if neonatal disease is left untreated include syphilitic chondritis and rhinitis (causes **saddle-nose deformity**), pathologic fractures, **bowing of the tibia** (= SABER SHIN), **V-shaped incisors** (= HUTCHINSON'S TEETH), multicuspid molars (= MULBERRY MOLARS), interstitial keratitis, and deafness.
Micro Pathology	N/A
Treatment	Penicillin.
Discussion	*Treponema pallidum* is a spirochete; in utero vertical transmission occurs from an infected mother to the fetus. Occurs maximally during 16–36 weeks of gestation; may be the cause of stillbirth. Preventable if the mother has received adequate treatment. **FIRST AID** p.187

. . . .

SYPHILIS - CONGENITAL

ID/CC	An 18-year-old white male presents with a **painless ulcer** on his **penis.**
HPI	He admits to having had **unprotected intercourse** with a prostitute three weeks ago.
PE	**Painless, single, rounded, firm papule with well-defined margins on dorsal aspect of glans penis that ulcerates** (= "HARD CHANCRE"); nontender, rubbery bilateral inguinal lymphadenopathy.
Labs	Treponemes on **dark-field examination** of exudate from chancre; VDRL positive; **FTA-ABS positive;** ELISA for HIV negative.
Imaging	N/A
Gross Pathology	A 1.2-cm ulcerated papule with rolled edges and induration; regional lymphadenopathy.
Micro Pathology	Capillary dilatation with plasma cell, PMN, and macrophage infiltration; fibroblastic reaction.
Treatment	**Benzathine penicillin** IM, 2.4 MU single dose.
Discussion	An STD caused by *Treponema pallidum*, a spirochete, it is characterized by the appearance of a painless chancre in the area of inoculation. If left untreated, secondary and tertiary syphilis may ensue. Other STDs, such as AIDS, are more prevalent in patients with syphilis. **FIRST AID** p.187

. . . .

SYPHILIS - PRIMARY

ID/CC	A 23-year-old female presents with a **nonpruritic skin eruption, hair loss,** and generalized fatigue and weakness.
HPI	She admits to having had **multiple sexual partners** and **unprotected sex.** She has had two spontaneous abortions.
PE	Extensive **raised, copper-colored, maculopapular, desquamative rash on palms and soles;** generalized nontender **lymphadenopathy** with hepatosplenomegaly; large, pale, **coalescent, flat-topped papules and plaques** in groin (= CONDYLOMATA LATA); dull, erythematous **mucous patches in mouth;** hair loss (= ALOPECIA) in tail of eyebrows.
Labs	Skin lesions, mucous patches in mouth, and condylomata lata positive for **treponemes; positive VDRL; positive FTA-ABS;** ELISA negative for HIV; CSF VDRL negative.
Imaging	N/A
Gross Pathology	N/A
Micro Pathology	N/A
Treatment	IM benzathine **penicillin.**
Discussion	**Sexual partners must be treated.** **FIRST AID** p.187

ID/CC	A 12-year-old white male presents with **stiffness of the jaw** and neck along with inability to swallow.
HPI	Twelve days ago he stepped on a **rusty nail,** which produced a small **puncture wound;** the area is now red, hard, and swollen with pus. He has been experiencing tingling sensations and spasms in his calf muscles. He has not received any immunizations within the past 10 years.
PE	**Jaw muscle rigidity** (= TRISMUS); **facial muscle spasm** (= RISUS SARDONICUS); **dysphagia; neck rigidity;** normal deep tendon reflexes; profuse sweating; patient alert, apprehensive, restless, and hyperactive during PE; loud noise elicits **painful spasms** of face, neck, abdomen, and back, the latter producing **opisthotonos.**
Labs	CBC, CSF, blood chemistries normal.
Imaging	N/A
Gross Pathology	There may be fractures of ribs or vertebrae with sustained spasms.
Micro Pathology	N/A
Treatment	**Surgical debridement of wound;** tetanus immune globulin intramuscularly or intrathecally; diazepam; phenobarbital; tetanus toxoid; penicillin IV.
Discussion	Caused by **tetanospasmin,** a neurotoxin produced by *Clostridium tetani,* an obligate anaerobic, spore-forming, gram-positive rod; the toxin blocks the release of the inhibitory neurotransmitter glycine in the anterior horn cells. Tetanus often occurs in IV drug abusers; neonates of nonimmunized mothers may become infected through the **umbilical cord stump.** The disease may occur even **years** after injury or infection and may also involve the autonomic nervous system (arrhythmias, high/low blood pressure).

∅ gly

TETANUS

ID/CC	A 40-year-old male diagnosed with **AIDS** presents with a **severe headache**.
HPI	He suffered a grand mal seizure two hours before his arrival in the emergency room. He denies any past history of seizures and adds that he has many pets, including **cats**.
PE	**Generalized lymphadenopathy;** bilateral **papilledema;** left-sided hemiparesis with hyperactive deep tendon reflexes on left side; positive Babinski's sign on left side.
Labs	Positive indirect fluorescent antibody test for toxoplasmosis; positive Sabin–Feldman dye test.
Imaging	MR/CT-Head: single or multiple rounded **mass lesions with ring or nodular enhancement.**
Gross Pathology	Large brain abscesses with concomitant focal neurologic abnormalities, seizures, or altered mental status.
Micro Pathology	Parasites appear in tissue as tachyzoites or encysted bradyzoites; aggregates of nonencapsulated organisms constitute pseudocysts.
Treatment	Pyrimethamine; sulfadiazine.
Discussion	The **intermediate host** of *Toxoplasma gondii* is the **cat**. Also transmitted by ingestion of raw or undercooked meat.

toxoplasmosis Rx: pyramethamine sulfadiazine

. . . .

TOXOPLASMOSIS

ID/CC	A 50-year-old man presents with generalized **myalgia** and a persistent **low-grade fever.**
HPI	In addition, the patient recalled having severe **abdominal pain and diarrhea several weeks ago.** The patient worked in a **pig slaughterhouse** for many years.
PE	VS: fever. PE: periorbital and facial edema; tenderness over calf, thigh, and shoulder muscles; conjunctival and splinter hemorrhages; no neurologic deficit seen.
Labs	CBC: **eosinophilia.** Normal ESR; **elevated serum CPK, LDH, and AST;** latex agglutination test positive for *Trichinella.*
Imaging	N/A
Gross Pathology	Facial, neck, biceps, lower back, and diaphragm most frequently affected muscles.
Micro Pathology	Biopsy of sternocleidomastoid muscle reveals cysts of *Trichinella spiralis.*
Treatment	Thiabendazole; high-dose corticosteroids.
Discussion	The organism causing the disease, *Trichinella spiralis*, can be transmitted when **raw or undercooked pork** is ingested.

Strongyloides

ID/CC A 12-year-old white male is brought to his pediatrician because of an **ulcer** on his right wrist together with **swelling of the lymph nodes** in the right axillae with **suppuration.**

HPI He had just returned from summer camp and, upon questioning, admits to having played with **rabbits** at the camp's breeding grounds. He has been suffering from **fever,** headache, and muscle aches for almost one week.

PE VS: fever. PE: indurated erythematous nodule with ulcer formation on right wrist; right axillary adenopathy with pus formation; lymphangitis; mild splenomegaly; scattered rales in both lung bases.

Labs CBC: **normal WBC count. Increased ESR;** elevated C-reactive protein; positive agglutination test; *Francisella tularensis* on direct fluorescent antibody staining of material from ulcer.

Imaging CXR: bilateral basilar interstitial infiltrates.

Gross Pathology Enlarged, indurated lymph nodes with necrosis and suppuration; skin nodule at site of inoculation with ulcer formation.

Micro Pathology Necrosis and suppuration of lymph nodes; pulmonary and disseminated lesions; **granulomatous nodules** with central caseating necrosis.

Treatment Streptomycin and tetracycline.

Discussion An acute zoonosis caused by *Francisella tularensis*, a nonmotile, aerobic, gram-negative bacillus; transmitted through contact with rabbits, squirrels, or other rodents or tick bites. It may be ulceroglandular, tonsillar, oculoglandular, pneumonitic, or typhoidal.

. . . .

TULAREMIA

ID/CC	A 27-year-old male is admitted to the hospital for evaluation of **increasing fever** of unknown origin along with malaise, headache, sore throat, cough, and **constipation.**
HPI	He visited Southeast Asia three weeks ago but did not receive any prior vaccinations.
PE	VS: **bradycardia**; fever; **fever charting reveals "stepladder" pattern.** PE: mild hepatosplenomegaly; faint **erythematous macules seen over trunk** (= "ROSE SPOTS").
Labs	CBC: neutropenia with relative lymphocytosis. **Widal's test** positive in significant titers; blood and stool cultures reveal *Salmonella typhi*.
Imaging	N/A
Gross Pathology	Infection of Peyer's patches in terminal ileum leads to necrosis of underlying mucosa, producing longitudinal oval ulcerations.
Micro Pathology	Ulcers bordered by mononuclear cells; typhoid nodules with lymphocytes and macrophages may be present in liver, spleen, and lymph nodes.
Treatment	Ciprofloxacin is curative.
Discussion	Because infection is acquired from contaminated food or water, typhoid vaccine is recommended for all those traveling to areas that have had typhoid epidemics. Two vaccines are available: a parenteral vaccine and a more recently licensed oral vaccine.

TYPHOID FEVER (ENTERIC FEVER)

ID/CC	A 5-year-old male presents with malaise, anorexia, fever, and a **pruritic rash on his scalp,** face, and trunk.
HPI	He also complains of a headache. Six of his **classmates** recently missed school because of **similar symptoms.**
PE	VS: fever (39 C). PE: skin lesions consist of **macules, papules, vesicles, pustules, and scabs, all present at same time,** predominantly over trunk, face, and scalp.
Labs	Multinucleated giant cells on scraping samples from vesicles. CBC: **leukopenia.**
Imaging	N/A
Gross Pathology	Macular, papular, vesicular, and pustular rash with scab formation; characteristically, all lesions present at same time (vs. variola); **lesions appear in crops** every 3–5 days; myocarditis and pneumonitis may be present.
Micro Pathology	Intranuclear, acidophilic inclusion bodies (= LIPSCHÜTZ BODIES) in epithelial cells with clear halo around them and multinucleated giant cells on histologic exam of skin lesions (on **Tzanck smear**).
Treatment	Acetaminophen; antihistamines and calamine lotion; hygienic measures, including isolation.
Discussion	A highly contagious dermotropic viral disease caused by varicella–zoster virus, a DNA herpesvirus, it is transmitted by direct contact. Complications include secondary bacterial infection of the skin and pneumonia; high-risk individuals may be protected passively with immunoglobulin.

. . . .

VARICELLA ZOSTER -CHICKENPOX

ID/CC	A 45-year-old **HIV-positive** male is seen by his family doctor following the appearance of a **painful, burning skin rash** on the **left side of his chest** that is accompanied by a headache and low-grade fever.
HPI	The patient had chickenpox as a child. He had been well until one year ago, when he was diagnosed with **non-Hodgkin's lymphoma,** for which he is currently undergoing **chemotherapy.**
PE	Vesicular rash on erythematous base; in **dermatomal distribution** (left T6–T8); exquisitely tender to touch.
Labs	Acantholytic cells on **Tzanck smear** from base of **vesicles.**
Imaging	N/A
Gross Pathology	N/A
Micro Pathology	Intranuclear eosinophilic inclusions surrounded by clear halo (= COWDRY A INCLUSIONS).
Treatment	Acyclovir.
Discussion	Reactivation of latent infection with **varicella–zoster virus;** the rash typically follows the distribution of a nerve root. It is commonly seen in **immunosuppressed patients** and is also associated with trauma, ultraviolet radiation, hypothermia, and **emotional stress.** Postherpetic neuralgia is a common complication in the elderly.

ID/CC   A 2-year-old female is brought to the emergency room because of **paroxysms** and multiple **coughs** in a single expiration, followed by a high-pitched **inspiratory whistle or whoop.**

HPI   For the past two weeks she has had a runny nose, low-grade fever, muscle pains, and headache. Her **immunization schedule is incomplete.**

PE   VS: fever. PE: child apprehensive and becomes cyanotic during cough paroxysm; thick green mucus expelled with cough; conjunctival injection.

Labs   CBC: **marked leukocytosis with lymphocytosis.** *Bordetella pertussis* on fluorescent antibody staining of nasopharyngeal secretions; diagnosis confirmed by culture on Bordet–Gengou medium.

Imaging   N/A

Gross Pathology   Small conjunctival and brain hemorrhages may appear during paroxysms; bronchiectasis may also be a complication.

Micro Pathology   Signs of acute inflammation in upper respiratory tract mucosa, with erythema, petechiae, polymorphonuclear infiltrate, and necrosis. → *mycoplasma*

Treatment   Largely supportive; **erythromycin.**

Discussion   A bacterial infection of the upper respiratory tract caused by *Bordetella pertussis*, a gram-negative coccobacillus, it is transmitted by droplets and comprises a prodromal (catarrhal), a paroxysmal, and a convalescent stage. Largely preventable with universally administered diphtheria, tetanus toxoid, and pertussis (DTP) vaccine. Pertussis toxin is a heat-labile exotoxin in which ADP ribosylates the inhibitory G protein, thus inactivating it and leading to constant activation of adenylate cyclase and increased cAMP.

↑ cAMP

· ·

WHOOPING COUGH

ID/CC	A 24-year-old white South American male develops sudden **high fever,** chills, generalized aches and pains, retro-orbital headache, nausea, and vomiting.
HPI	He gradually improves, but the fever returns four days later along with a **yellowing of his skin and eyes** and an episode of fainting and abundant **coffee-ground emesis.**
PE	VS: **fever** (39 C); hypotension (BP 90/60). PE: **jaundice;** petechiae on lower legs; swollen, bleeding gums; cardiomegaly; hepatomegaly.
Labs	CBC: **leukopenia.** UA: oliguria; **albuminuria;** hematuria.
Imaging	N/A
Gross Pathology	Normal-sized liver with yellowish hue and petechiae; pale, swollen kidneys.
Micro Pathology	Characteristic **midzonal lobular necrosis,** fatty accumulation, and eosinophilic intracytoplasmic Councilman bodies on liver biopsy; hyperplasia of endothelial cells surrounding lymphoid follicles of spleen; **severe renal tubular damage** with epithelial fatty degeneration and necrosis.
Treatment	Symptomatic; prevention with mosquito control and live viral vaccination.
Discussion	A viral hemorrhagic fever caused by a flavivirus transmitted by *Aedes* **mosquitoes;** preventable by a vaccine, which is required prior to travel to certain countries. It is associated with a mortality rate of 5%–10%, but most cases are self-limiting and mild. Similar to malaria but does not recur.

· ·

YELLOW FEVER

ID/CC	A 50-year-old white male develops **sudden fever with chills,** pain in the back and extremities, and **neck stiffness;** he vomited six times and had a **convulsion** prior to admission.
HPI	The patient is a **heavy smoker** and is **diabetic. Two weeks ago,** he had a **URI.** He is also very sensitive to light (= PHOTOPHOBIA).
PE	Markedly reduced mental status (= OBTUNDED); petechial rash over trunk and abdomen; **nuchal and spinal rigidity; positive Kernig's and Brudzinski's signs;** no focal neurologic deficits.
Labs	LP: **elevated pressure; cloudy CSF; elevated protein; markedly decreased glucose; high cell count with mostly WBCs.** CSF Gram stain reveals **gram-positive diplococci.**
Imaging	CT/MR-Brain: **meningeal thickening** and enhancement.
Gross Pathology	Pia–arachnoid congestion results from inflammatory infiltrate; thin layer of pus forms and promotes adhesions while obstructing normal CSF flow (can cause hydrocephalus); brain covered with purulent exudate, most heavily on base.
Micro Pathology	N/A
Treatment	IV antibiotics; penicillin. *rifampin prophylax*
Discussion	A pyogenic infection of the CNS that requires prompt treatment. *S. pneumoniae* is the most common cause of adult meningitis.

. . . .

BACTERIAL MENINGITIS - ADULT

ID/CC	A **4-year-old** female presents with a one-week history of **fever,** severe **headache, irritability,** and **malaise; two** days ago she developed **neck stiffness,** and her parents report **projectile vomiting** over the past 24 hours.
HPI	The child is also very sensitive to light (= PHOTOPHOBIA). She is fully immunized and has no history of ear, nose, and throat infection, skin rashes, dog bites, or foreign travel.
PE	VS: fever. PE: irritability; resistance to being touched or moved; minimal papilledema of fundus; no focal neurologic signs; no cranial nerve deficits; positive **Kernig's** and **Brudzinski's** signs.
Labs	CBC: **neutrophilic leukocytosis.** LP: increased pressure; **cloudy CSF; neutrophilic pleocytosis; decreased glucose; increased protein; gram-negative coccobacilli.** Negative ZN and India ink staining; normal serum electrolytes; on chocolate agar, blood culture grew *H. influenzae;* negative Mantoux.
Imaging	CT/MR-Brain: **meningeal thickening** and enhancement.
Gross Pathology	Abundant accumulation of purulent exudate between pia mater and arachnoid; meningeal thickening; cloudy to frankly purulent CSF.
Micro Pathology	Intense neutrophilic infiltrate.
Treatment	IV antibiotics; consider steroids.
Discussion	A pyogenic infection of the nervous system primarily affecting the meninges, it is most commonly caused by pneumococcus (*S. pneumoniae,* associated with sickle cell anemia), meningococcus (*Neisseria meningitidis*, associated with a petechial skin rash), and *H. influenzae* (most commonly in children). Less commonly caused by enterobacteria, *Streptococcus* species, *Staphylococcus* species (due to dental infection), and anaerobic organisms (due to trauma).

. . . .

BACTERIAL MENINGITIS - PEDIATRIC

ID/CC A 33-year-old **HIV-positive** white male is brought into the emergency room by his mother because of a **persistent headache.**

HPI The patient's mother states that her son has been suffering for a long time from **headaches** and **stiff neck** as well as from fever and chills.

PE VS: fever (39 C). PE: **severe nuchal rigidity;** lack of responsiveness to any command; positive **Kernig's** and **Brudzinski's** signs; diminished patellar and Achilles reflexes; clear lung sounds.

Labs LP: increased CSF pressure; variable pleocytosis (75 lymphocytes/mm^3); elevated protein; decreased glucose. **Heavily encapsulated, nondimorphic spherical fungal cells** (= *CRYPTOCOCCUS NEOFORMANS*) **revealed on India ink staining;** polysaccharide capsular antigen detected on latex agglutination test; diagnosis confirmed by culture on Sabouraud's medium.

Imaging CT/MR-Brain: **multiple ring-enhancing lesions.**

Gross Pathology Granuloma and abscess formation, mainly at base of brain; CNS primarily affected; lungs affected less commonly.

Micro Pathology Abundant fungi in CSF and leptomeninges, with slight mononuclear inflammatory reaction; typical **nodular granulomatous meningitis** with exudate.

Treatment Amphotericin B and 5-flucytosine; fluconazole.

Discussion Once called torulosis, cryptococcosis is the most common cause of mycotic meningitis; it is acquired through the inhalation of dried **pigeon droppings** and is usually seen in **immunocompromised patients.**

· ·

CRYPTOCOCCAL MENINGITIS

ID/CC	A 30-year-old homosexual white male presents to his family physician with a **rapidly progressive diminution of vision.**
HPI	He is known to be **HIV positive** and periodically comes in for checkups.
PE	**Cotton-wool exudates, necrotizing retinitis, and perivascular hemorrhages** on funduscopic exam.
Labs	N/A
Imaging	N/A
Gross Pathology	N/A
Micro Pathology	N/A
Treatment	Ganciclovir; foscarnet (CMV is resistant to acyclovir).
Discussion	CMV retinitis is an important **treatable cause of blindness** that occurs in 20% of AIDS patients. Toxoplasmosis and progressive multifocal leukoencephalopathy (PML) are other important causes of blindness in AIDS patients.

· ·

CYTOMEGALOVIRUS (CMV) RETINITIS

ID/CC A 43-year-old male **Mexican** migrant worker visits his ophthalmologist because of pain and **loss of vision** in his right eye.

HPI Recently he has also suffered from **severe headaches** and **projectile vomiting.**

PE **Papilledema** on left funduscopic exam; **free-floating cyst** in vitreous body of right eye; chorioretinitis and disk hemorrhage; multiple nontender subcutaneous nodules.

Labs CBC: eosinophilia. LP: lymphocytic and eosinophilic pleocytosis in CSF with elevated protein and decreased glucose. Eggs of *Taenia solium* in stool sample.

Imaging XR-Plain: small nodular calcifications. CT/MR-Brain: characteristic ring-enhancing **intracranial** cysts or calcifications; can cause obstruction and hydrocephalus.

Gross Pathology Fluid-filled cysts containing scolex surrounded by fibrous capsule in anterior chamber of eye; intraventricular and parenchymal invasion of brain, subcutaneous tissue, and striated muscle.

Micro Pathology Inflammatory infiltration of cyst by PMNs; necrotic inflammation with calcification upon death of parasite.

Treatment Surgical removal of parasite from eye; albendazole, corticosteroids/praziquantel for brain disease.

Discussion Produced by *Cysticercus cellulosae*, the larval form of the pork tapeworm *Taenia solium*, it is due to the ingestion of ova and spreads through fecal–oral transmission.

· ·

NEUROCYSTICERCOSIS

ID/CC	A 3-year-old male, the child of recent African immigrants, is brought to the local health center because of **asymmetrical legs.**
HPI	His parents give a history of **incomplete immunization.** They add that five months ago the boy had **fever and diarrhea** that subsided spontaneously; a few weeks later they noted that he could not use his right leg.
PE	Right leg **thin, short, wasted, weak, and flaccid; absent deep tendon reflexes** in right leg; **no sensory deficit;** upper limbs normal; mental status and cranial nerves normal.
Labs	EMG: chronic partial denervation with abnormal spontaneous activity in resting muscle and reduction in number of motor units under voluntary control; normal sensory conduction studies.
Imaging	N/A
Gross Pathology	N/A
Micro Pathology	N/A
Treatment	Rehabilitation, supportive.
Discussion	A symptomatic disease caused by poliovirus that is more common in infants and children, it can result in muscular atrophy and skeletal deformity. Attacks anterior horn cells and may affect cranial nerves (bulbar polio); preventable by vaccine.

ID/CC   A 54-year-old man presents with **ataxia, mental status changes,** grossly **deformed ankle joints,** and **shooting pains in his extremities.**

HPI   He remembers having had a "boil" on his penis (= PRIMARY SYPHILITIC CHANCRE) many years ago that went away by itself. He also recalls having had a scaling rash on the soles of his feet and the palms of his hands (due to secondary syphilis) some time ago.

PE   Painless **subcutaneous granulomatous nodules** (= GUMMAS); **reduced joint position and vibration sense in both lower extremities** (due to bilateral dorsal column destruction); loss of deep tendon reflexes in both lower limbs; loss of pain sensation and **deformed ankle and knee joints with effusion** (= CHARCOT'S NEUROPATHIC ARTHROPATHY); **broad-based gait;** positive Romberg's sign (due to sensory ataxia); **pupillary light reflex lost but accommodation reflex retained** (= ARGYLL ROBERTSON PUPILS).

Labs   Positive VDRL and *Treponema pallidum* hemagglutination assay (TP-HA). **LP: pleocytosis and increased proteins in CSF;** VDRL positive. Normal blood glucose levels.

Imaging   CXR: "tree-bark calcification" of ascending aorta.

Gross Pathology   Obliterative endarteritis and meningoencephalitis.

Micro Pathology   Proliferation of microglia; demyelinization and axonal loss in dorsal roots and columns.

Treatment   Penicillin.

Discussion   **Tabes dorsalis** usually develops 15–20 years after initial infection. There may also be visceral involvement (can cause neurogenic bladder).

ID/CC	A 25-year-old woman visits her family physician because of marked **burning pain while urinating** (= DYSURIA), **increased frequency of urination** with **small amounts of urine** (= POLLAKIURIA), and passage of a few drops of **blood-stained** debris at the end of urination (= HEMATURIA).
HPI	She got married two weeks ago and has **just returned from her honeymoon.**
PE	VS: no fever; normotension. PE: no edema; no costovertebral angle tenderness; moderate suprapubic tenderness with **urgency.**
Labs	UA: urine collected in two glasses; second glass more turbid and blood-stained; urine sediment reveals RBCs and WBCs; **no RBC or WBC casts;** Gram stain of urine sediment reveals **gram-negative bacilli;** *E. coli* in significant colony count (> 100,000) on urine culture.
Imaging	N/A
Gross Pathology	N/A
Micro Pathology	N/A
Treatment	Oral antibiotics; adequate hydration.
Discussion	*E. coli* is the most common pathogen; *Proteus, Klebsiella, Staphylococcus saprophyticus,* and *Enterococcus* are other common bacteria causing cystitis. Hemorrhagic cystitis may result from adenoviral infection.

· ·

ACUTE CYSTITIS

ID/CC A 28-year-old black woman who is in her 27th week of pregnancy complains of **right flank pain, high-grade fever,** malaise, headache, and **dysuria.**

HPI Thus far her pregnancy has been uneventful.

PE VS: fever. PE: no peripheral edema; **right costovertebral angle tenderness; acutely painful fist percussion on right lumbar area** (= POSITIVE GIORDANO'S SIGN).

Labs CBC: leukocytosis with neutrophilia. UA: proteinuria; hematuria; abundant WBCs and **WBC casts;** pyocytes on sediment; alkaline pH; **urine culture > 100,000 colonies** of *E. coli.*

Imaging US-Renal: slightly enlarged kidney.

Gross Pathology Kidney enlarged, edematous, and hyperemic with microabscesses in medulla.

Micro Pathology Pyocytes in tubules; **light blue neutrophils on supravital stain** (= GLITTER CELLS); PMN infiltration of interstitium.

Treatment Antibiotics according to sensitivity; ampicillin; in nonpregnant patients, an aminoglycoside may be added as initial treatment.

Discussion An acute bacterial kidney infection caused mainly by gram-negative bacteria such as *E. coli, Klebsiella, Proteus, and Enterobacter;* usually results from upward dissemination of lower urinary tract bacteria.

· ·

ACUTE PYELONEPHRITIS

ID/CC	A 19-year-old male goes to his health clinic complaining of **painful urination and discharge.**
HPI	The patient had **casual sex with a classmate** while at a party **two weeks ago.** He has had no previous STDs.
PE	Watery yellowish-green discharge from meatus; no penile ulcerations or inguinal lymphadenopathy.
Labs	**Numerous neutrophils but no bacteria** on Gram stain of discharge; **positive** direct immunofluorescence using monoclonal **antibody against *Chlamydia;*** routine bacterial cultures, including Thayer–Martin, do not show growth.
Imaging	N/A
Gross Pathology	N/A
Micro Pathology	N/A
Treatment	Tetracycline; **doxycycline;** azithromycin; treat both patient and sexual partner.
Discussion	The most common cause of nongonococcal urethritis is *Chlamydia trachomatis*; less frequently caused by *Ureaplasma urealyticum.* It is frequently coincident with gonococcal urethritis.

NONGONOCOCCAL URETHRITIS

ID/CC   A 15-year-old male presents with **painful bilateral swelling of the parotid glands,** left-sided scrotal pain, and fever.

HPI   Nothing in the patient's history suggests that he had childhood mumps. He has not received a measles-mumps-rubella (MMR) vaccination.

PE   VS: fever. PE: bilateral parotid gland enlargement with obliteration of mandibular hollow; hyperemia and edema of Stensen's duct (parotid duct) orifice; retroauricular lymphadenopathy; left-sided scrotal and **testicular swelling with tenderness.**

Labs   CBC: leukopenia with **lymphocytosis; hyperamylasemia.** *pancreatitis* Positive complement fixation antibodies; positive serologic enzyme immunoassay (EIA) for mumps antibody (repeat test after one week to demonstrate a fourfold rise).

Imaging   US-Scrotum: increased color flow and edema.

Gross Pathology   Enlarged, edematous testicle.

Micro Pathology   Parotid glands show perivascular mononuclear, lymphocytic, and plasma cell infiltrate with necrosis; ductal obstruction and edema; testicular interstitial edema; perivascular cerebral lymphocytic cuffing.

Treatment   Scrotal support; analgesics, ice packs; corticosteroids.

Discussion   Orchitis may be caused by bacterial infections such as *E. coli* and other enterobacteria; viral infections such as **mumps;** STDs such as *Chlamydia* species or gonorrhea; or pathogens such as *Mycobacterium tuberculosis*. Mumps orchitis may give rise to sterility if bilateral.

· ·

ORCHITIS

ID/CC	A 25-year-old **sexually active female** complains of **burning on urination.**
HPI	She also complains of pain in the lower abdomen and **increased frequency of urination.**
PE	Mild suprapubic tenderness.
Labs	UA: mild proteinuria; hematuria; WBCs but no casts seen. Urine culture reveals > **100,000** *E. coli* organisms present.
Imaging	N/A
Gross Pathology	Infection ascends the urinary tract (urethritis, cystitis, pyelonephritis); mucosal hyperemia and edema.
Micro Pathology	Urothelial hyperplasia and metaplasia.
Treatment	Ciprofloxacin. bactrim
Discussion	Eighty percent of UTIs are caused by *E. coli*; *Staphylococcus saprophyticus* is the second most common cause. Other causes, in order of frequency, are *Proteus, Klebsiella, Enterobacter, Serratia, Pseudomonas,* and *Enterococcus*; *Chlamydia* and *Neisseria* are also causes of urethritis. Risk factors include female gender, sexual activity, pregnancy, obstruction, bladder dysfunction, vesicoureteral reflux, and catheterization. **FIRST AID** p.191

· ·

URINARY TRACT INFECTION (UTI)

From the authors of *Underground Clinical Vignettes*

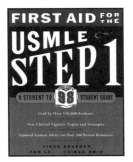

A true classic used by over 200,000 students around the world. The '99 edition features details on the new computerized test, new color plates and thoroughly updated high-yield facts and book reviews. Bi-directional links with the *Underground Clinical Vignettes Step 1* series. ISBN 0-8385-2612-8.

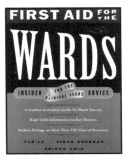

This high-yield student-to-student guide is designed to help students make the transition from the basic sciences to the hospital wards and succeed on their clinical rotations. The book features an orientation to the hospital environment, tips on being an effective and efficient junior medical student, student-proven advice tailored to each core rotation, a database of high-yield clinical facts, and recommendations for clinical pocket books, texts, and references. ISBN 0-8385-2595-4.

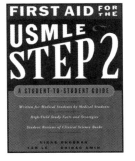

This entirely rewritten second edition now follows in the footsteps of *First Aid for the USMLE Step 1*. Features an exam preparation guide geared to the new computerized test, basic science and clinical high-yield facts, color plates and ratings of USMLE Step 2 books and software. Bi-directional links with the *Underground Clinical Vignettes Step 2* series.

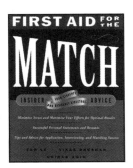

This top rated (5 stars, *Doody Review*) student-to-student guide helps medical students effectively and efficiently navigate the residency application process, helping them make the most of their limited time, money, and energy. The book draws on the advice and experiences of successful student applicants as well as residency directors. Also featured are application and interview tips tailored to each specialty, successful personal statements and CVs with analyses, current trends, and common interview questions with suggested strategies for responding. ISBN 0-8385-2596-2.

The *First Aid* series by Appleton & Lange...the review book leader.
Available through your local health sciences bookstore !

About the Authors

. . . .

VIKAS BHUSHAN, MD
Vikas is a diagnostic radiologist in Los Angeles and the series editor for *Underground Clinical Vignettes*. His interests include traveling, reading, writing, and world music. He is single and can be reached at vbhushan@aol.com

CHIRAG AMIN, MD
Chirag is an orthopedics resident at Orlando Regional Medical Center. He plans on pursuing a spine fellowship. He can be reached at chiragamin@aol.com

TAO LE, MD
Tao is completing a medicine residency at Yale-New Haven Hospital and is applying for a fellowship in allergy and immunology. He is married to Thao, who is a pediatrics resident. He can be reached at taotle@aol.com

JOSE M. FIERRO, MD
Jose (Pepe) is beginning a med/peds residency at Brookdale University Hospital in New York. He was a general surgeon in Mexico and worked extensively in Central Africa. His interests include world citizenship and ethnic music. He is married and can be reached at jmfierro@aol.com

HOANG NGUYEN
Hoang (Henry) is a third-year medical student at Northwestern University. Henry is single and lives in Chicago, where he spends his free time writing, reading, and enjoying music. He can be reached at hbnguyen@nwu.edu

VISHAL PALL, MBBS
Vishal recently completed medical school and internship in Chandigarh, India. He hopes to begin his Internal Medicine residency training in the US in July 1999. He can be reached at vishalpall@hotmail.com